CHILDREN'S ISSUES, LAWS AND PROGRAMS

CHILD FATALITIES DUE TO MALTREATMENT

THE ROLE OF QUALITY DATA

CHILDREN'S ISSUES, LAWS AND PROGRAMS

Additional books in this series can be found on Nova's website under the Series tab.

Additional E-books in this series can be found on Nova's website under the E-books tab.

SOCIAL ISSUES, JUSTICE AND STATUS

Additional books in this series can be found on Nova's website under the Series tab.

Additional E-books in this series can be found on Nova's website under the E-books tab.

CHILDREN'S ISSUES, LAWS AND PROGRAMS

CHILD FATALITIES DUE TO MALTREATMENT

THE ROLE OF QUALITY DATA

VERNON CHAPMAN
AND
ALLAN BURTON
EDITORS

New York

For permission to use material from this book please contact us:
Telephone 631-231-7269; Fax 631-231-8175
Web Site: http://www.novapublishers.com

Library of Congress Cataloging-in-Publication Data

Child fatalities due to maltreatment : the role of quality data / editors, Vernon Chapman and Allan Burton.
p. cm.
Includes index.
ISBN 978-1-61942-342-8 (soft cover)
1. Child abuse--United States. 2. Child abuse--Reporting--United States. 3. Children--Mortality--United States. 4. Child welfare--United States. I. Chapman, Vernon, 1973- II. Burton, Allan, 1976-
HV6626.52C558 2011
362.760973--dc23
2011045825

Published by Nova Science Publishers, Inc. † New York

CONTENTS

PREFACE

Children's deaths from maltreatment are especially distressing because they involve a failure on the part of adults who were responsible for protecting them. Questions have been raised as to whether the federal National Child Abuse and Neglect Data System (NCANDS), which is based on voluntary state reports to the Department of Health and Human Services (HHS), fully captures the number of circumstances of child fatalities from maltreatment. This book examines the extent to which HHS collects and reports comprehensive information on child fatalities from maltreatment and looks to strengthen data quality, expand available information, improve sharing, and estimate better the costs and benefits of collecting national data on near fatalities.

Chapter 1 - Children's deaths from maltreatment are especially distressing because they involve a failure on the part of adults who were responsible for protecting them. Questions have been raised as to whether the federal National Child Abuse and Neglect Data System (NCANDS), which is based on voluntary state reports to the Department of Health and Human Services (HHS), fully captures the number or circumstances of child fatalities from maltreatment. GAO was asked to examine (1) the extent to which HHS collects and reports comprehensive information on child fatalities from maltreatment, (2) the challenges states face in collecting and reporting this information to HHS, and (3) the assistance HHS provides to states in collecting and reporting data on child maltreatment fatalities. GAO analyzed 2009 NCANDS data—the latest data available—conducted a nationwide Web-based survey of state child welfare administrators, visited three states, interviewed HHS and other officials, and reviewed research and relevant federal laws and regulations.

Chapter 2 - I serve as the Director of the National Center for the Review and Prevention of Child Deaths, formerly known as the National Center for Child Death Review. We are based at the Michigan Public Health Institute. We are a resource center beginning our tenth year, funded through a cooperative agreement with the Maternal and Child Health Bureau within the Health Resources and Services Administration at HHS. Our center provides training and technical assistance to states as they work to conduct comprehensive and multidisciplinary case reviews of child deaths. Child Death Review (CDR) expanded to most states in the late 1990s, through training support from the Administration on Children and Families and OJJDP at the Department of Justice. In 2003, HRSA established funds for our national resource center, to encourage the focus on the prevention of deaths through the reviews. Today every state and Washington DC, with the exception of Idaho, has a CDR program in place but states vary greatly in their CDR structures, administrative homes, funding levels, and timing of reviews. Forty-four states have legislation requiring reviews and there is no national legislation requiring or supporting CDR. CAPTA legislation does however encourage death reviews of children known to the child welfare system through the citizen review process. Thirty-seven states support reviews at the county level with a state level advisory board that reviews these local findings to improve state policy and practice. Twelve states only have state-level review teams. Most states review deaths from a wide variety of causes including diseases, accidents, homicides and suicides-but all states review deaths from child abuse and neglect. All states review deaths from birth to age 18. There are two U. S. Healthy People 2020 Objectives especially related to CDR: *allstates and the District of Columbia will review 100% of allsudden and unexpected infant deaths and all deaths from external causes*-this would include child maltreatment.

Chapter 3 - It is one in which I have been involved for 40 years, including the time that I served as Maine's health and human services commissioner, and while at the Child Welfare League of America.

According to official federal statistics, 13,856 children died from child abuse and neglect during the 2001-2009 period. Additionally, several studies have concluded there actually is significant undercounting of maltreatment deaths, and that the true number may be several thousands more than reported.

Much can be done to reduce these child abuse and neglect deaths. There exists a vast body of knowledge about healthy child growth and development, including how to prevent abuse in the first place, and how to protect children from further harm if abuse should occur. But the sheer amount of child abuse and neglect in America—already more than 20 million reports of maltreatment made to government agencies in this decade—is certain evidence that, despite the best efforts of the many who work daily to address this problem, we continue to fall far short in applying our knowledge.

While the day to day direct responsibility for the protection of at-risk children rests with thousands of local and state child protection agencies, law enforcement, and courts across the country, their efforts could be greatly strengthened by expanding federal planning, coordination, and funding aimed at reducing child deaths.

Chapter 4 - I thank you for the opportunity to testify on child deaths due to maltreatment. I am a Professor of Pediatrics at Brown Medical School and the Director of the Child Protection Program at Hasbro Children's Hospital in Providence, Rhode Island. I have provided medical care for abused and neglected children for over 28 years. I have a unique perspective on this issue because I believe I am the only person in this room who has often stood at the bedside in the emergency department or in the intensive care unit and actually witnessed the deaths of infants and children from maltreatment.

When the death of a child is a result of abuse or neglect, a sad event becomes an immense tragedy.[1] This was certainly seen most recently in the public outcry over the death of Kaylee Anthony, a previously healthy, happy toddler.

Chapter 5 - I have worked in the child welfare arena for more than a decade. In 1998, I left my civil litigation practice and started working as an attorney for the Children's Law Center in Los Angeles (CLC-LA) representing thousands of children over my tenure there. After working at CLC-LA for almost six years, I became interested in taking my experience working with children and families and translating it into systemic improvement. I earned a PhD in policy analysis at the Pardee RAND Graduate School, writing my dissertation on improving outcomes for teenage mothers in the child welfare system. After receiving my PhD in 2008, I came to work at the Center for Public Policy Priorities, a non-profit, nonpartisan think tank based in Austin, Texas that is committed to improving public policy to better the economic and social condition of low- to moderate-income Texans. At the Center, I work on child welfare policy and budget issues. I conduct research, participate in state and national coalitions and educate policy makers on how to create better outcomes for children and families.

In: Child Fatalities Due to Maltreatment
Editors: V. Chapman and A. Burton
ISBN: 978-1-61942-342-8

Chapter 1

CHILD MALTREATMENT: STRENGTHENING NATIONAL DATA ON CHILD FATALITIES COULD AID IN PREVENTION[1]

United States Government Accountability Office

WHY GAO DID THIS STUDY

Children's deaths from maltreatment are especially distressing because they involve a failure on the part of adults who were responsible for protecting them. Questions have been raised as to whether the federal National Child Abuse and Neglect Data System (NCANDS), which is based on voluntary state reports to the Department of Health and Human Services (HHS), fully captures the number or circumstances of child fatalities from maltreatment. GAO was asked to examine (1) the extent to which HHS collects and reports comprehensive information on child fatalities from maltreatment, (2) the challenges states face in collecting and reporting this information to HHS, and (3) the assistance HHS provides to states in collecting and reporting data on child maltreatment fatalities. GAO analyzed 2009 NCANDS data—the latest data available—conducted a nationwide Web-based survey of state child welfare administrators, visited three states, interviewed HHS and other officials, and reviewed research and relevant federal laws and regulations.

[1] This is an edited, reformatted and augmented version of the Congressional Research Service Report, dated July 2011.

What GAO Recommends

GAO recommends that the Secretary of HHS take steps to further strengthen data quality, expand available information on child fatalities, improve information sharing, and estimate the costs and benefits of collecting national data on near fatalities. In its comments, HHS agreed with GAO's findings and recommendations and provided technical comments, which GAO incorporated as appropriate.

What GAO Found

More children have likely died from maltreatment than are counted in NCANDS, and HHS does not take full advantage of available information on the circumstances surrounding child maltreatment deaths. NCANDS estimated that 1,770 children in the United States died from maltreatment in fiscal year 2009. According to GAO's survey, nearly half of states included data only from child welfare agencies in reporting child maltreatment fatalities to NCANDS, yet not all children who die from maltreatment have had contact with these agencies, possibly leading to incomplete counts. HHS also collects but does not report some information on the circumstances surrounding child maltreatment fatalities that could be useful for prevention, such as perpetrators' previous maltreatment of children. The National Center for Child Death Review (NCCDR), a nongovernmental organization funded by HHS, collects more detailed data on circumstances from 39 states, but these data on child maltreatment deaths have not yet been synthesized or published.

States face numerous challenges in collecting child maltreatment fatality data and reporting to NCANDS. At the local level, lack of evidence and inconsistent interpretations of maltreatment challenge investigators—such as law enforcement, medical examiners, and child welfare officials—in determining whether a child's death was caused by maltreatment. Without medical evidence, it can be difficult to determine that a child's death was caused by abuse or neglect, such as in cases of shaken baby syndrome, when external injuries may not be readily visible. At the state level, limited coordination among jurisdictions and state agencies, in part due to confidentiality or privacy constraints, poses challenges for reporting data to NCANDS.

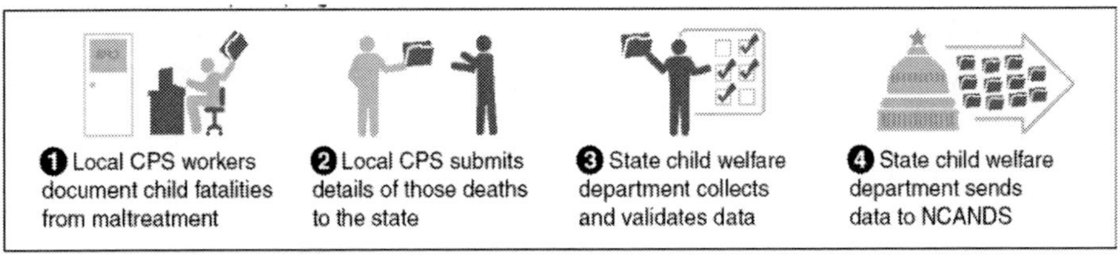
1 Local CPS workers document child fatalities from maltreatment
2 Local CPS submits details of those deaths to the state
3 State child welfare department collects and validates data
4 State child welfare department sends data to NCANDS

Source: GAO analysis of site visit information.

General Process for Reporting Child Maltreatment Fatalities That Are Known to Child Protective Service (CPS) Agencies to NCANDS.

HHS provides assistance to help states report child maltreatment fatalities, although states would like additional help. For example, HHS hosts an annual NCANDS technical assistance conference, provides individual state assistance, and, through NCCDR, has developed resources to help states collect information on child deaths. However, there has been limited collaboration between HHS and NCCDR on child maltreatment fatality information or prevention strategies to date. State officials indicated a need for additional information on how to coordinate across state agencies to collect more complete information on child maltreatment fatalities. States are also increasingly interested in collecting and using information on near fatalities from maltreatment.

ABBREVIATIONS

AAP	American Academy of Pediatrics
ABA	American Bar Association
ACF	Administration for Children and Families
CAPTA	Child Abuse Prevention and Treatment Act
CDC	Centers for Disease Control
CDR	Child Death Review
CFSR	Child and Family Services Review
CPS	child protective services
CRS	Congressional Research Service
DOJ	Department of Justice
EVAA	Enhanced Validation and Analysis Application
FBI	Federal Bureau of Investigation
HHS	Department of Health and Human Services

HIPAA	Health Insurance Portability and Accountability Act
HRSA	Health Resources and Services Administration
NCANDS	National Child Abuse and Neglect Data System
NCCDR	National Center for Child Death Review
NCHS	National Center for Health Statistics
NCIPC	National Center for Injury Prevention and Control
NDACAN	National Data Archive on Child Abuse and Neglect
NIS	National Incidence Study of Child Abuse and Neglect
NRC	National Resource Center
NRC-CWDT	National Resource Center for Child Welfare Data and Technology
OMB	Office of Management and Budget
SDC	summary data component
SIDS	sudden infant death syndrome
SUID	sudden unexplained infant death

July 7, 2011

The Honorable Dave Camp
Chairman
Committee on Ways and Means
House of Representatives

Dear Mr. Chairman:

Every year, children in the United States die after being physically abused, severely neglected, or otherwise maltreated, frequently at the hands of their parents or others who are entrusted with their care. Infants and toddlers are the most vulnerable to such abuse and neglect. According to estimates by the National Child Abuse and Neglect Data System (NCANDS), 1,770 children in the United States died from physical abuse or other forms of maltreatment in fiscal year 2009.[1] Some experts believe that more children have died from maltreatment than are captured in these estimates. Additionally, experts expressed concern that national data on these deaths may be problematic for understanding the issue because of inconsistencies and limitations in the data collected and reported to NCANDS by states. In addition, many more children are severely harmed and may nearly die from maltreatment, but NCANDS does not collect data specifically on near fatalities. Collecting complete and consistent information is important for understanding the magnitude of the problem and for targeting efforts to help prevent future child deaths and near deaths from maltreatment.

The Department of Health and Human Services (HHS) is the principal federal agency that provides oversight of state child welfare systems, which are intended, in part, to protect children who have been maltreated and help prevent maltreatment. To better understand the scope of child maltreatment, including child fatalities,[2] and inform efforts to address and prevent it, the 1988 amendments to the Child Abuse Prevention and Treatment Act (CAPTA) required HHS to establish a national data collection and analysis program for child maltreatment data.[3] HHS responded to this mandate by establishing and maintaining NCANDS, which is a voluntary data-reporting system. Since at least 2000, states have increasingly provided data on children who were maltreated to HHS for NCANDS. From these data, HHS publishes a yearly *Child Maltreatment* report. The most recent report, for fiscal year 2009, presents national data about child abuse and neglect known to child welfare agencies in the United States. As of fiscal year 2009, all states reported at least some data on child maltreatment to NCANDS.

To obtain more information about the quality of national data on child fatalities and near fatalities from maltreatment, the Chairman, House Ways and Means Committee, asked us to examine (1) the extent to which HHS collects and reports comprehensive information on child fatalities from maltreatment, (2) the challenges states face in collecting and reporting information on child fatalities from maltreatment to HHS, and (3) the assistance HHS provides to states in collecting and reporting data on child fatalities from maltreatment.

We used multiple methodologies to address these three objectives. For the first objective, we reviewed published research on the number of child fatalities and systematically assessed the adequacy of each study's research methodology. We analyzed fiscal year 2009 NCANDS data provided to HHS by states and additional data on child maltreatment fatalities collected from states by a nongovernmental organization funded by HHS, the National Center for Child Death Review. We confirmed the reliability of these data for our purposes. We also interviewed HHS officials responsible for NCANDS child maltreatment data, child welfare practitioners, and other experts. We conducted a nationwide Web-based survey of state child welfare administrators in 50 states, the District of Columbia, and Puerto Rico between October and December 2010.[4] We received survey responses from all states, although not all states responded to every question. To address the second objective, we conducted site visits to California, Michigan, and Pennsylvania to obtain a more in-depth understanding of states' child fatality data issues in addition to drawing upon the state survey.[5] To address the third objective, we interviewed HHS NCANDS officials and other experts, analyzed survey results on states' perspectives on additional NCANDS assistance needed from HHS, and reviewed HHS technical assistance and other documents relevant to child maltreatment fatalities and near fatalities. We also reviewed CAPTA and implementing regulations and federal guidance on collecting and reporting maltreatment data, as well as other related laws, including pertinent state laws. (See app. I for additional information on our scope and methodology.)

We conducted this performance audit from April 2010 through July 2011 in accordance with generally accepted government auditing standards. Those standards require that we plan and perform the audit to obtain sufficient, appropriate evidence to provide a reasonable basis for our findings and conclusions based on our audit objectives. We believe that the evidence obtained provides a reasonable basis for our findings and conclusions based on our audit objectives.

BACKGROUND

About 53,000 children died from a range of causes in the United States in 2007—the latest year for which national data were available—according to the Centers for Disease Control and Prevention (CDC).[6] Major causes of death among children include conditions originating in the perinatal period, accidents (such as motor vehicle traffic accidents and drowning), congenital anomalies, homicide, and cancer.[7] Of all children who died in fiscal year 2009, NCANDS estimates that 1,770 children died from various types of maltreatment.[8] (See figure 1.) Moreover, 81 percent of children who died from maltreatment were 3 years old or younger, and more than half were infants 1 year or younger.

According to NCANDS, the estimated number of child maltreatment fatalities has increased nationally over the past 5 years, from 1,450 in fiscal year 2005 to 1,770 in fiscal year 2009. HHS reported that states believe this increase may be due, in part, to new state legislation, new procedures, and improved state reporting practices.

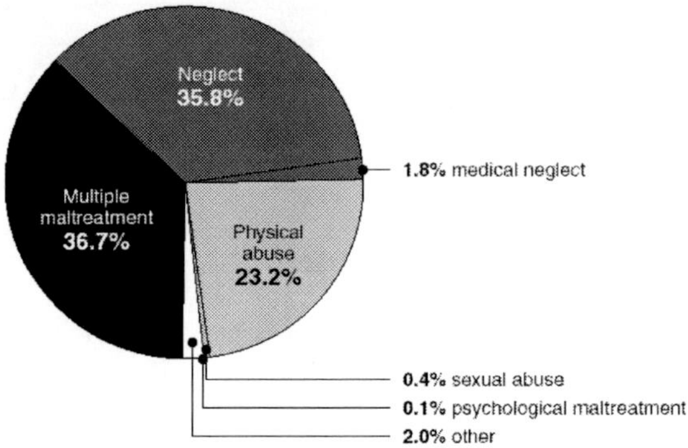

Source: Data from HHS *Child Maltreatment 2009* report.

Note: This analysis is based on 1,343 child deaths reported by 44 states through child-specific, case-level data. Because of this, the total number is smaller than the 1,770 NCANDS estimate for child fatalities from maltreatment. Fatalities can be attributed to more than one type of maltreatment.

Figure 1. Child Fatalities by Type of Maltreatment, Fiscal Year 2009.

Protecting children from maltreatment is primarily the responsibility of child welfare programs administered at the state and local levels. In all states, child protective services (CPS) are part of the child welfare system.[9] CPS generally screens and responds to suspected child maltreatment reported to it by mandatory reporters—including police officers, doctors, teachers, and other professionals—as well as by neighbors and family members. In fiscal year 2009, professionals initiated 58 percent of all reports of suspected maltreatment to CPS. CPS investigators determine whether such reports are considered maltreatment under state laws or policies.[10] CPS also typically determines whether interventions—such as placement with a foster family—are in the best interest of the child. When CPS determines that a child's death is from maltreatment, CPS documents the case. The state's child welfare department reports it to NCANDS.[11] (See figure 2.)

At the federal level, most of the $8.4 billion in federal assistance dedicated to child welfare purposes ($7.2 billion) in fiscal year 2010 supports state child welfare programs, including foster care, adoption assistance, and child protection. HHS oversees funding provided to states that support child welfare programs, and provides technical assistance and training to states on a variety of child welfare issues. HHS has a technical assistance contract specific to NCANDS and also provides technical assistance on NCANDS and other data issues through its National Resource Centers (NRC).[12]

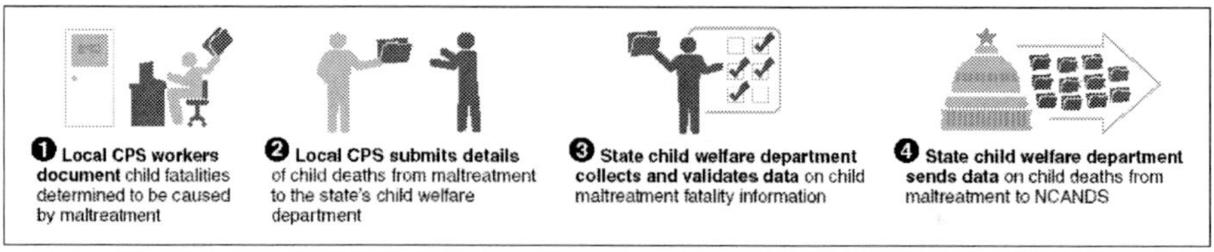

Source: GAO analysis of site visit information.

Figure 2. General Process for Reporting Child Maltreatment Fatalities Known to CPS to NCANDS.

CAPTA is the key federal legislation focused on preventing and responding to child maltreatment. Reauthorized in 2010, CAPTA provides supports for, among other things, data collection activities and technical assistance on child maltreatment.[13] It also authorizes federal funding to states for grants to support prevention, investigation, and treatment of child maltreatment. In fiscal year 2010, funding for CAPTA programs totaled about $97 million, of which $26.5 million was for basic state grants to improve CPS. These grants are distributed to states by formula,[14] and may be used to improve CPS investigations, caseworker training, and prevention programs. All states in fiscal year 2010 received CAPTA basic state grants. To receive this grant, states are required to have an approved state plan that outlines the activities that the state intends to implement. It must include, for example, provisions or procedures for receiving and responding to allegations of child abuse or neglect and for ensuring children's safety. For grant purposes, child abuse and neglect is defined as "at a minimum, any recent act or failure to act on the part of a parent or caretaker, which results in death, serious physical or emotional harm, sexual abuse or exploitation, or an act or failure to act which presents an imminent risk of serious harm."[15]

Each state receiving a basic grant is also required to establish and support citizen review panels to evaluate the effectiveness of CPS policies, procedures, and practices, and, according to the National Center for Child Death Review, 14 states in 2003 reported that their child death review teams serve a dual function as CAPTA citizen review panels for child fatalities. The citizen review panels must be composed of volunteers who are "broadly representative" of the community, including members with expertise in the prevention and treatment of child abuse and neglect, and may include members of foster care review boards or child death review teams.[16] Child death review teams exist in all but one state to review child abuse and neglect fatalities and suspicious child deaths. Results of these reviews may be used to improve services, advocate for change, and conduct public awareness activities, ultimately for the purpose of preventing future child maltreatment deaths.

Near Fatalities of Children from Maltreatment

CAPTA defines the term “near fatality” as “an act that, as certified by a physician, places the child in serious or critical condition.”[17] Although the term is defined, neither CAPTA nor the applicable regulations further discuss data collection on near fatalities. NCANDS does not have a specific data field that identifies the case as a near fatality from maltreatment.[18]

Child Maltreatment Data Collected by NCANDS

NCANDS collects and analyzes data on children involved in situations in which CPS either investigated an allegation of maltreatment or initiated an alternative response. State CPS agencies generally are responsible for submitting NCANDS data to HHS. Since 1996, states that receive basic state grants under CAPTA have been required to report annually—”to the maximum extent practicable”—at least 12 data items to NCANDS on child maltreatment.[19]

Data from NCANDS are an important source of information for several publications, reports, and activities of the federal government, as well as for child welfare officials, researchers, and others. NCANDS data are compiled annually in the *Child Maltreatment* report, which, as of December 2010, has been issued annually since 1992. HHS issues the annual *Child Welfare Outcomes: Report to Congress* partly based on state submissions of NCANDS data. This report presents information to Congress on states’ performance on national child welfare outcomes, including NCANDS data on reducing the recurrence of child maltreatment and reducing child maltreatment in foster care. NCANDS data have also been incorporated into the Child and Family Services Reviews (CFSR).[20] Finally, NCANDS data are used to help assess the performance of several HHS programs in accordance with the Program Assessment Rating Tool.

National Data Likely Underestimate the Number of Children Who Died from Maltreatment and Provide Incomplete Information on Circumstances

More Children Have Likely Died from Maltreatment than Are Counted in National Data

More children have likely died from maltreatment than are reflected in the national estimate of 1,770 child fatalities for fiscal year 2009. According to our survey, child welfare officials in 28 states thought that the official number of child maltreatment fatalities in their state was probably or possibly an undercount. Child welfare experts and HHS officials we spoke with also thought that national estimates did not reflect the full extent of children's deaths from maltreatment and that undercounting was an issue with child fatalities. Acknowledging the limitations of NCANDS data on child maltreatment fatalities, HHS's *Child Maltreatment 2009* report states that NCANDS fatality data are only a proportion of all child fatalities caused by maltreatment. These data are based on reports provided to NCANDS by CPS agencies within state child welfare departments.[21]

A major reason for the likely undercounting of child maltreatment fatalities is that nearly half of states report to NCANDS data only on children already known to CPS agencies—yet not all children who die from maltreatment were previously brought to the attention of CPS.[22] Some children may not have been previously maltreated, or their earlier maltreatment may not have been noticed or reported to CPS agencies.[23] Child deaths from maltreatment are recorded in many state and local data sources, such as death certificates from state vital statistics offices and medical examiner or coroner's offices, CPS records, and state and local child death review team records (see figure 3),[24] and in Federal Bureau of Investigation (FBI) Uniform Crime Reports at the federal level.

Because of this, HHS also attempts to capture the fatalities of maltreated children who were not previously known to state CPS agencies. Specifically, HHS instructs states on how to report data from non-CPS agencies and encourages states to obtain information on child maltreatment fatalities from other state agencies.[25] However, in responding to our survey, 24 states reported that their 2009 NCANDS data did not include child fatality information from any non-CPS sources.[26] More specifically, for example, 43 states responded that their NCANDS data did not include child fatality data from the vital statistics department. (See figure 4.) Since NCANDS is a voluntary data-reporting system, state CPS agencies cannot be required to obtain information from other state agencies, according to HHS officials.

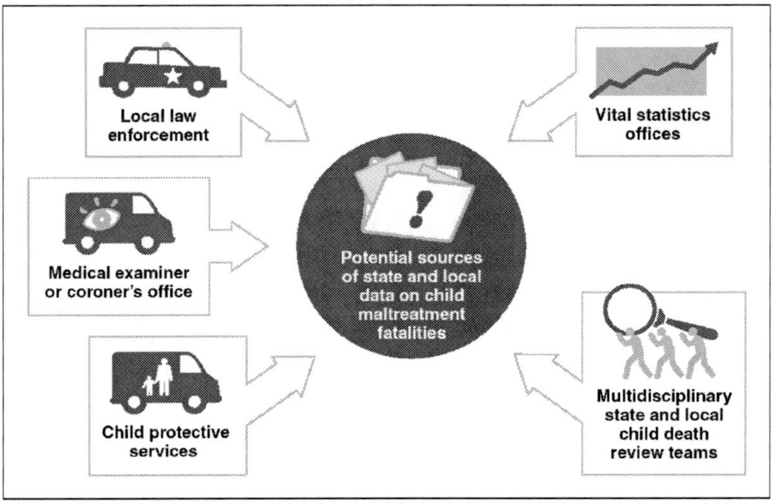

Source: GAO analysis of state survey data.

Figure 3. Potential Sources of State and Local Data on Child Maltreatment Fatalities.

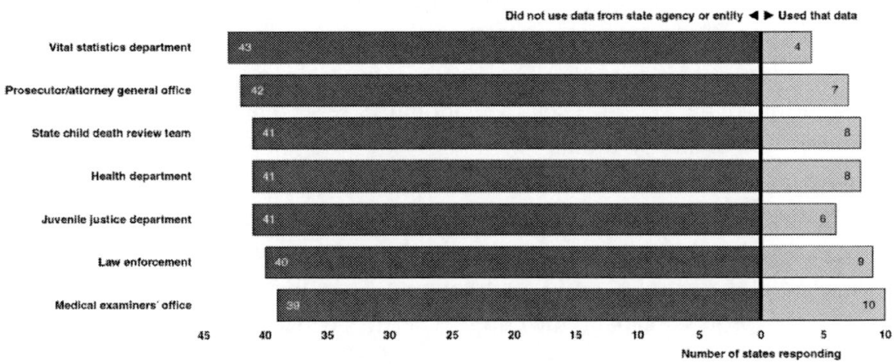

Source: GAO analysis of state survey data.

Note: Data reflect state child welfare officials' responses to question about data reported to NCANDS through the agency file. The total number of states responding varies by item number.

Figure 4. State Child Welfare Agencies That Did and Did Not Use Information from External Sources for Reporting Child Fatalities to NCANDS.

Synthesizing information about child fatalities from multiple sources can produce a more comprehensive picture of the extent of child deaths than sole reliance on CPS data. In our review of research assessing whether the number of child fatalities from maltreatment was accurate, we found that key sources of information undercounted child deaths, sometimes by significant amounts.[27] For example, a peer-reviewed study of fatal child maltreatment in three states found that state child welfare records undercount child fatalities from maltreatment by from 55 percent to 76 percent.[28] The data sources analyzed in this study were death certificates, state child welfare agency records, state child death review team data, and law enforcement reports to the FBI Uniform Crime Report system. The study found that each data source reviewed undercounted the total number of child maltreatment fatalities. However, more than 90 percent of the child fatality cases could be identified by linking any two of the data sources, demonstrating the value of using multiple existing data sources to determine the extent of child fatalities from maltreatment. The study also found that the multidisciplinary child death review team process may be the most promising approach to identifying deaths from maltreatment if there is a standardized data collection and reporting system in place.

Using a different methodology, HHS's most recent National Incidence Study of Child Abuse and Neglect (NIS-4)—issued in January 2010—estimated 2,400 child deaths from maltreatment in the study year spanning portions of 2005 and 2006.[29] The NIS is a congressionally mandated, periodic effort of HHS to estimate the incidence of child abuse and neglect in the United States.[30] Unlike NCANDS, which relies primarily on CPS data reported by states, the NIS-4 relies on multiple sources of child death information. The NIS-4 used a nationally representative sample of 122 counties to create national estimates of the incidence, severity, and demographic distribution of child maltreatment, including fatalities from maltreatment. The NIS-4 uses two standardized research definitions of maltreatment in developing its findings.[31] In each county, NIS-4 collected CPS data as well as reports of child maltreatment cases that came to the attention of community professionals in the county sheriff's office; the county departments of juvenile probation, health, and public housing; municipal police departments; hospitals; public schools; day care centers; shelters; and voluntary social services and mental health agencies.[32]

Furthermore, several factors complicate the ability to obtain comprehensive information on child fatalities from maltreatment. As a result, it can be difficult to compare child fatality data across states or over time.

Table 1. Differing State Definitions of Medical Neglect

Definition of medical neglect	States using this definition
Failing to provide any special medical treatment or mental health care needed by the child	Mississippi, North Dakota, Ohio, Oklahoma, Tennessee, Texas, and West Virginia
Withholding medical treatment or nutrition from disabled infants with life-threatening conditions	Indiana, Kansas, Minnesota, and Montana

Source: HHS analysis of state laws in use as of July 31, 2009.

- **Inconsistent definitions of maltreatment:** Although CAPTA legislation establishes a minimum standard for the definition of child abuse and neglect, states generally develop their own variations of these definitions.[33] Consequently, child maltreatment data at the national level can reflect an underlying inconsistency across individual states. For example, some states add medical neglect to the CAPTA definition and define the concept differently. (See table 1.) Some experts we interviewed said that definitions need to be standardized nationally to improve the quality of NCANDS data.[34] When states submit data to NCANDS, HHS requires them to align state definitions of child maltreatment with elements of the NCANDS definitions, using a data-mapping process.[35] HHS officials told us this mapping process helps create more consistent data within NCANDS. However, the mapping process may not fully address underlying state differences in determining whether a child's death was regarded as a maltreatment death. HHS officials told us they considered definitional variations less important as a factor affecting NCANDS data quality than the difficulty in obtaining agreement among various local and state investigators—such as law enforcement and medical personnel—that maltreatment was the cause of a child's death.
- **Differing legal standards for substantiating maltreatment:** Because states have different legal standards for substantiating maltreatment, it is difficult to compare data across states. The substantiation process generally requires child welfare caseworkers to decide whether an allegation of maltreatment, or the risk of maltreatment, meets the criteria established by state law or policy. In a Congressional Research Service (CRS) analysis, state standards for substantiating child maltreatment were categorized into three groups,

ranging from least to most rigorous. CRS found that states with stricter standards for substantiating maltreatment have the lowest rates of child maltreatment. (See table 2.)

- **Missing data:** Some states do not report any information on child fatalities in certain years (e.g., Alaska, Massachusetts, and North Carolina for fiscal year 2009). Additionally, some states do not report particular data elements. For example, in fiscal year 2009, 13 states did not report information on children who died who, within the past 5 years, had been in foster care and had been reunited with their families;[36] 7 states did not report the relationship of the perpetrator to the child who died; and 6 states did not report the race or ethnicity of the child who died. In responding to our survey, states provided a range of explanations for missing data in their NCANDS submissions. For example, according to state child welfare officials, key reasons for their not reporting some data were that other state entities, not child welfare, collected the information; state data systems did not collect those data; and delays occurred in data collection that affected reporting.

Table 2. States' Use of Standards of Evidence for Substantiation of Maltreatment

Level of evidence required for investigator to substantiate child abuse or neglect	Number of states with given level of evidence	Victim rate (Victims per 1,000 children in given states) in fiscal year 2007
Least strict		
Credible (or reasonable determination) that a child had been abused or neglected.	20	13.3
More strict		
Preponderance of evidence supported a determination that a child was a victim of abuse or neglect.	28	9.4
Strictest		
Clear and convincing evidence that a child had been abused or neglected.	2	1.7

Source: Congressional Research Service analysis based on data provided in HHS, *Child Maltreatment 2008*.

- **Lack of death date:** NCANDS does not ask states to identify the date of a child's death, and establishing maltreatment as the cause of a child's death can take many months, particularly when a criminal proceeding is involved. As a result, child deaths reported to NCANDS may have, in fact, occurred earlier than the year in which they are reported.

HHS Collects but Does Not Report Some Useful Information on the Circumstances Surrounding Child Fatalities

NCANDS collects more data on the circumstances surrounding child fatalities than are reflected in HHS's annual *Child Maltreatment* report—information that could be useful for prevention.[37] NCANDS collects information from state CPS agencies about the demographics of children who died, such as their age and race; the report of maltreatment and the CPS agencies' response and investigation; the perpetrator; services provided to the family; and risk factors associated with the child and with the caretaker.[38] It also collects information on broad categories of maltreatment—such as neglect, physical abuse, sexual abuse, psychological maltreatment, and medical neglect—although it does not collect more detailed information on how a child dies, such as from a bathtub incident or swimming pool drowning resulting from a parent's neglect.[39] However, HHS does not report some information it collects on the circumstances surrounding child fatalities.[40] For example, when we analyzed unpublished fiscal year 2009 state data reported to NCANDS on children's deaths from maltreatment, we found the following:

- **Types of abuse:** Rates of physical abuse were slightly higher among older children who died from maltreatment (ages 8 to 18), while neglect rates were slightly higher among younger children who died from maltreatment (ages 7 and younger).
- **Child welfare history:** At least 14 percent of children who died from maltreatment had a previous substantiated or indicated incident of child maltreatment.[41]
- **Perpetrators:**[42]
  - Sixteen percent of perpetrators of fatal child maltreatment were previously involved in an incident of child maltreatment that was either substantiated or indicated by CPS.

    - Among parents who were perpetrators, about 60 percent were female. Of unmarried partners who were perpetrators, 90 percent were male.[43]
- **Child's risk factors:** Two percent of maltreated children who died had a disability such as a developmental disability, an intellectual disability, or a visual or hearing impairment.[44]

According to experts, detailed information on the circumstances surrounding child fatalities can provide a more comprehensive understanding of the issue of fatal child maltreatment, such as revealing patterns that could aid prevention efforts.

In addition to what is known nationally through NCANDS data, extensive information on the circumstances surrounding children's deaths from maltreatment is collected by the Child Death Review Case Reporting System (CDR Reporting System), operated by the nongovernmental National Center for Child Death Review (NCCDR).[45] NCCDR serves as a resource center for state and local multidisciplinary teams that review cases of child deaths for the purpose of improving case identification, investigations, services, follow-up, and prevention.[46] Nearly all states have child death review teams comprising CPS workers, prosecutors, law enforcement, coroners or medical examiners, public heath care providers, and others.[47] While data received from NCCDR are more detailed in each case, the data are less comprehensive than those reported to NCANDS, according to HHS. Local review teams do not review all cases of possible death due to maltreatment but rather vary in their roles and scope from locality to locality. NCCDR is funded largely by the Maternal and Child Health Bureau of the Health Resources and Services Administration (HRSA).[48]

Begun in 2005, NCCDR's Web-based CDR Reporting System is potentially a rich source of multistate data on child fatalities from all causes, including child maltreatment.[49] As of June 1, 2011, 39 states had data use agreements with NCCDR, according to NCCDR officials. NCCDR's goal is to eventually have all state child death review teams provide information on child fatalities to the data system, according to these officials. NCCDR takes a public health approach to child death review, with a focus on improving investigations and identifying modifiable risk factors and strategies for preventing similar future deaths. According to NCCDR, most states using the system analyze their data and publish annual reports. Although NCCDR conducts in-house analyses for federal partner organizations, such as the National Highway Traffic Safety Administration, according to NCCDR officials, or of sudden cardiac deaths for a hospital, CDR data on child maltreatment deaths have not yet been synthesized or published, according to the NCCDR director.[50] (The sidebar describes the CDR data-reporting form.)

NCCDR's Child Death Review Case Reporting Form

NCCDR developed the Child Death Review Case Reporting Form to collect comprehensive information on child fatalities from state and local teams that conduct child death reviews. This case reporting form was developed in cooperation with 30 state child death review leaders and advocates. The case reporting form documents detailed information about the circumstances involved in the child's death, such as the manner of death (e.g., homicide or accident), the cause of death (e.g., injury or neglect), the child welfare history of children who die from maltreatment, the investigative actions taken, services provided or needed, and key risk factors. The system collects comprehensive information on the history of the child, primary caregivers, supervisors, and perpetrators of acts of omission and/or commission. It also collects further details about the method of death (such as by fire, weapon, asphyxia, poisoning, or drowning) and collects details on subtypes of physical abuse deaths (e.g., abusive head trauma, chronic battered child syndrome, beating, scalding, or burning) and neglect deaths (e.g., failure to protect from hazards, failure to provide necessities, failure to seek or follow treatment, or abandonment). The case reporting form collects information on actions recommended or taken by states' child death review teams to prevent similar deaths and improve agency systems. It also allows for the collection of information on near deaths of children as well as fatalities.

Source: GAO analysis of NCCDR information.

LOCAL INVESTIGATIVE CHALLENGES AND LIMITED COORDINATION HINDER STATES' EFFORTS TO COLLECT CHILD MALTREATMENT FATALITY DATA AND REPORT TO NCANDS

Investigative Difficulties Can Hamper Local Data Collection Efforts

Challenges faced by local investigators, such as law enforcement officials, medical examiners, and CPS staff, in determining whether a child's death was caused by maltreatment make it difficult for states to collect complete data on child maltreatment fatalities. These investigative challenges include lack of definitive medical evidence, limited resources for testing, differing expertise and training, and inconsistent interpretations and application of maltreatment definitions.

- **Lack of definitive medical evidence:** Without definitive medical evidence, it can be difficult to determine that a child's death was caused by abuse or neglect. According to our survey, 43 states indicated that medical issues were a challenge in determining child maltreatment.[51] (See figure 5.) For example, investigators we spoke with in California said that determining the cause of death in cases such as sudden unexplained infant death is challenging because the child may have been intentionally suffocated but external injuries are not readily visible. Similarly, a medical examiner we interviewed in Michigan said that it is a challenge to appropriately determine the cause of death for babies who may have been shaken to death or suffocated.[52] According to experts we spoke with, a lack of evidence also makes it difficult to determine whether a death was caused by neglect. Medical neglect is a type of maltreatment caused by failure of the caregiver to provide for the appropriate health care of the child despite having the resources—financial or otherwise—to do so.[53] Medical neglect often results from inattentiveness to a chronic illness or missing follow-up medical appointments, according to a physician from the American Academy of Pediatrics (AAP) Committee on Child Abuse and Neglect. For example, one expert told us that a medically fragile premature infant who is discharged from the hospital but not brought back in for a follow-up examination and later dies could be considered to have died from medical neglect. Experts from the American Bar Association's (ABA) Center on Children and the Law said neglect deaths are often categorized incorrectly, which may contribute to the problem of undercounting deaths from neglect. County officials we spoke with in Michigan added it is very difficult to determine medical neglect as the cause of death because the death can appear to have been from "natural" causes.

- **Limited resources for testing:** Another challenge in determining whether maltreatment was the cause of death is resource constraints that can limit the ability to conduct autopsies and medical tests. According to experts we spoke with from AAP, an autopsy provides much information on the factors contributing to a child's death—such as infection, trauma, or congenital heart disease—that cannot be determined based on visual inspection. These experts indicated that financial constraints of local and state governments are the primary reason autopsies are not conducted more regularly.[54] In Pennsylvania, a county coroner told us that even though autopsies can help clarify the cause and circumstances of a death, coroners have to make difficult choices in deciding when to order autopsies since they are expensive and there is limited funding to cover them. According to a 2009 report by the National Academy of Sciences, insufficient funding for testing influences cause-of-death determinations.[55] A law enforcement official we spoke with in Michigan noted that only 6 of his 20 requests for DNA testing were granted because of recent state cutbacks affecting crime laboratories. In our survey, 36 states identified limited resources as a challenge to identifying and investigating maltreatment deaths. (See figure 5.)
- **Differing expertise and training:** Differing levels of investigator expertise—particularly among those charged with determining the cause and manner of death—also present challenges to states in collecting child maltreatment fatality data. The National Academy of Sciences notes that the skill and training of coroners and medical examiners vary greatly. For example, in some counties, medical examiners—who are physicians and typically receive death investigation training—are charged with determining the cause and manner of death, including identifying maltreatment, while other counties rely on a coroner—who may or may not be a physician or have had any medical training—to make these determinations. A medical examiner and a coroner we spoke with in California noted

that because of differing expertise and training, forensic pathologists and medical examiners might categorize sudden infant deaths differently.[56] In 1996, CDC developed a protocol for sudden infant deaths in an effort to standardize reporting these deaths (see sidebar). While training can enhance skills for conducting maltreatment investigations, 35 states identified limited investigator training as a challenge in our survey. (See figure 5.) County officials in the three states we visited also told us that a lack of funding contributes to limited training opportunities. However, training opportunities were available in the states we visited. For example, state officials in California told us that all CPS staff are trained to recognize and report child abuse. County officials also said coroners in the state receive annual training that includes case presentations by investigators and forensic pathologists, which often include child deaths.[57]

CDC Sudden Unexplained Infant Death (SUID) Investigation Reporting Form

In 1996, CDC developed the SUID Investigation Reporting Form to establish a standard death scene investigation protocol for all sudden unexplained infant deaths. A revised version of this protocol, in addition to guidelines and training materials, is available on CDC's Web site, and some investigators use this tool to meet their data collection needs. The protocol guides investigators through the steps involved in an investigation, including questions to ask when interviewing witnesses, and provides a means to document findings. According to CDC, by standardizing data collection, this protocol improves the classification of SIDS and other unexplained infant deaths. Two of the three states we visited had standardized protocols—similar to CDC's SUID Reporting Form—for investigating sudden unexplained infant deaths. One of these states also had a standardized protocol for conducting autopsies that medical examiners and coroners use for infants whose deaths are sudden and unexplained.

Source: GAO analysis of information from CDC and California and Michigan site visits.

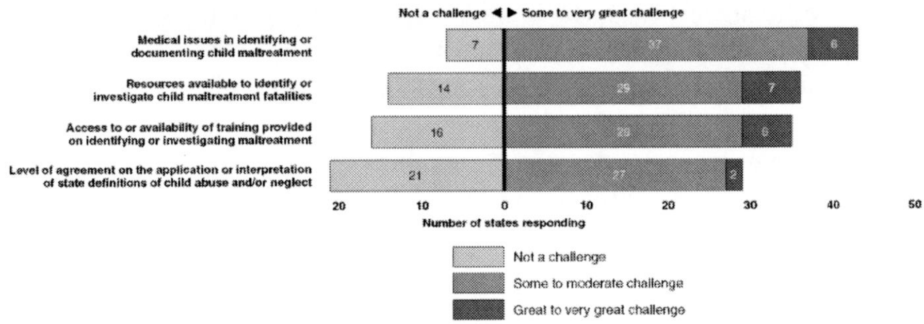

Source: GAO analysis of state survey data.

Figure 5. Challenges Investigators Face Identifying Child Maltreatment Fatalities.

- **Inconsistent interpretations and application of maltreatment definitions.** Differing interpretations and application of maltreatment definitions by investigators can lead to inconsistent determinations of cause of death. Law enforcement officials we spoke with in California noted that law enforcement officials and coroners sometimes disagree on the manner or cause of death, for example, when the death is suspected to be from natural causes but there is some indication of abuse or neglect. In our survey, 29 states indicated that the level of agreement among responsible entities—such as law enforcement officials, medical examiners or coroners, and CPS—about how to interpret and apply state definitions of child abuse or neglect was a challenge for collecting information on child maltreatment fatalities. (See figure 5.) These entities may use their own definitions and have different goals. For example, county officials in Michigan told us that law enforcement investigates for the purpose of determining probable cause for prosecution, while CPS investigates to determine if there is a preponderance of evidence for maltreatment. AAP experts stated that certain injuries—such as abusive head trauma—are often incorrectly categorized on child death certificates as natural or accidental when the real cause of death is abuse-related. It is also difficult to distinguish at autopsy between sudden infant death syndrome (SIDS) and accidental or deliberate suffocation with a soft object, according to the AAP.

  In our survey, 33 states indicated that variations across counties and other jurisdictions in identifying cause of death pose a challenge for collecting fatality information. For example, child death review team officials in Pennsylvania noted significant variability across counties in identifying child maltreatment deaths from head trauma. Similarly, state officials in California noted that some counties interpret co-sleeping deaths as maltreatment, while other counties do not, which creates inconsistencies in the numbers of child maltreatment deaths at the state level. Officials we interviewed in Michigan told us that when an external agency cross-checked its 2005 CPS data with medical records for 186 cases, the analysis indicated that 37 child deaths labeled as natural, accidental, or undetermined should have been documented as maltreatment. This variability across counties can result in greater data inconsistencies in states where the child welfare agency is county-administered with state supervision, as opposed to a state-administered system, according to national child welfare advocates. While 11 states indicated in our survey that their child welfare program was county- or locally administered, some of these states have large child populations, including California, New York, Ohio, and Pennsylvania.

Limited Coordination and Data Access Issues Pose Reporting Challenges

State child welfare officials indicated experiencing challenges coordinating among geographic jurisdictions within the state and across state lines. In our survey, 37 states indicated that the level of coordination among different jurisdictions poses a challenge for obtaining information on child maltreatment fatalities. (See figure 6.) For example, a local CPS official in Pennsylvania told us that it can be difficult for CPS to track children when families cross county lines. State officials we interviewed in Michigan also indicated that counties face challenges obtaining medical records and death certificates from jurisdictions in another state when children are taken across state borders to the nearest trauma center in the interest of providing immediate care.

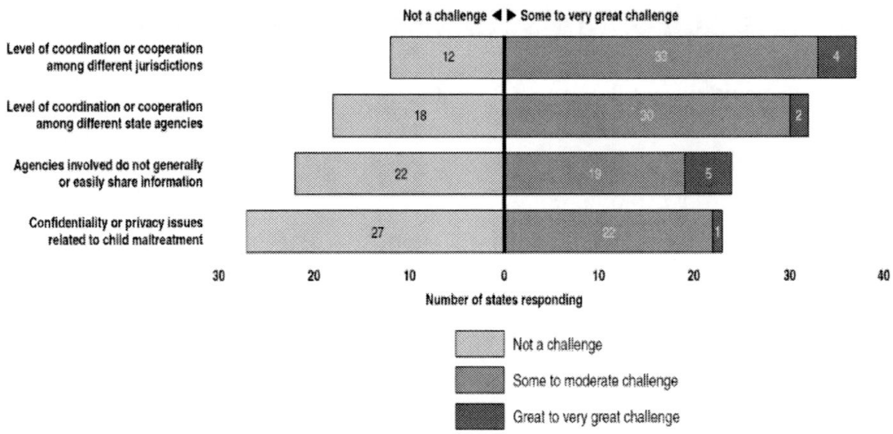

Source: GAO analysis of state survey data.

Figure 6. Challenges States Face Coordinating among Jurisdictions and Agencies.

States also indicated that limited coordination with other state agencies—particularly obtaining records from the health department—can challenge their ability to report information on child maltreatment fatalities to NCANDS. According to our survey, 32 states faced challenges coordinating among state agencies. Twenty-four states indicated that agencies involved in collecting information on child maltreatment fatalities do not generally or easily share information, and 23 states cited confidentiality or privacy issues related to child maltreatment as a challenge.[58] (See figure 6.) For example, child welfare officials in California told us their department had restricted data sharing with the department of public health after a security breach, and had only recently renewed its data-sharing agreement. Michigan officials specifically identified confidentiality and privacy restrictions as a challenge to obtaining child maltreatment fatality data because stakeholder agencies, such as the health department, are sometimes unsure what, if any, information they can share with child welfare. Furthermore, state officials in Pennsylvania told us that state and county child welfare officials are concerned about their limited access to records from drug and alcohol programs—which can include cases involving parents of a child who died—held by another state agency. California has coordinated across multiple agencies in an effort to produce a more accurate estimate of child maltreatment fatalities (see sidebar).

California's Reconciliation Audit

California uses a "reconciliation audit" to generate an estimate of child fatalities for NCANDS. The audit compares data from five sources—homicide files and child abuse central index files from the state department of justice, child welfare agency records, state department of health records, and files from county child death review teams. This audit is made possible by a state law that requires the state department of health to track child maltreatment deaths in California and requires multiple agencies to share data for the purpose of establishing accurate information on the nature and extent of these deaths (Cal. Penal Code § 11174.34 (Deering 2008)). According to the California official in charge of conducting the audit, the number of deaths estimated by this process is usually two-thirds higher than the number produced by any one data source. In the most recent audit, in 2008, the child welfare agency recorded 24 known cases of child maltreatment fatalities, but the reconciliation audit, which was submitted to NCANDS, found an estimated 185 cases.

Source: GAO analysis of California state information.

States indicated that several issues related to their data systems—especially those affecting electronic capabilities—have affected the completeness of child maltreatment fatality data they report to NCANDS. For example, although Pennsylvania collects certain CAPTA data elements, the state is unable to aggregate and report to NCANDS some of the information received from counties because this information is not recorded electronically, according to state officials. The inability to link different agencies' data systems with each other was also cited as a reporting challenge by 28 states. (See figure 7.) States also experienced challenges reporting to NCANDS when they were either converting from one data system to another or updating their current system. According to our survey, 9 states were challenged by piloting or implementing a new child welfare information system, and the *Child Maltreatment 2009* report shows that multiple states had incomplete or incomparable data because of system conversions. For example, Michigan was unable to submit data on child fatalities to NCANDS for fiscal year 2008, according to a state official, because of data errors associated with conversion

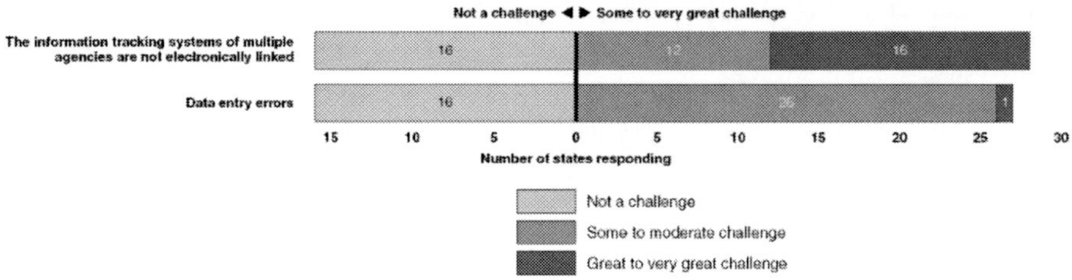

Source: GAO analysis of state survey data.

Figure 7. Challenges States Face with Data Systems.

to a new data system. In addition, 27 states responding to our survey reported that data entry errors posed a challenge for reporting child maltreatment fatality data to NCANDS. (See figure 7.)

To help mitigate these and other challenges, states are implementing quality controls on the child maltreatment fatality data they submit to NCANDS. According to our survey, 34 of the 50 states responding to this question indicated that their child welfare department had a quality control process—aside from HHS's Enhanced Validation and Analysis Application (EVAA), which assesses the quality of state data—to improve the accuracy of child maltreatment fatality data.

HHS Provides Assistance to States in Reporting on Child Maltreatment Fatalities, but States Would Like Additional Help

HHS Provides Technical Assistance to States in Reporting Data on Child Maltreatment

HHS provides assistance to states in several ways to help them report information on child maltreatment to NCANDS. NCANDS is supported by a technical team, composed of Children's Bureau and contractor staff, that provides technical assistance and tools to states for reporting child maltreatment fatality data. There is also an NCANDS State Advisory Group that worked closely with the technical team to design and implement NCANDS and now continues to meet annually to review and update NCANDS collection and reporting processes. According to HHS, this 20-member group helps ensure that enhancements to NCANDS accurately reflect states' experiences collecting data.[59] The NCANDS technical team also hosts the NCANDS Annual State Technical Assistance Meeting, a key means of assistance to states in which HHS officials provide NCANDS training and updates and states share questions and information. In 2010, child welfare representatives from 38 states participated in this 3-day meeting, which included workshops on data validation, error reporting, and methods for improving the quality of data provided to NCANDS. In our survey, 36 state officials reported that these annual NCANDS meetings were moderately helpful to very helpful. The NCANDS technical team has also developed Web-based resources with information and guidance to states on NCANDS data reporting, available through the NCANDS Web portal. The NCANDS portal is the key interface between states and the NCANDS technical team, and includes guidelines about reconciling and submitting data. The portal also contains an NCANDS Listserv where state officials can share information and obtain peer-to-peer assistance, according to HHS officials.

States can also obtain individualized NCANDS technical assistance upon request. Each state has an assigned NCANDS technical team liaison who can provide targeted information and support to help states report data to NCANDS. During the 2010 data-reporting process, all states were in communication with their NCANDS technical team liaisons, according to an NCANDS report. In our survey, state officials reported high levels of satisfaction with the technical teams' assistance, with 29 of the 50 states responding to this question identifying the help they received as moderately helpful to very helpful. State officials can also request on-site technical assistance regarding data collection and reporting from the National Resource Center for Child Welfare Data and Technology.[60]

HHS also provides assistance to states' child death review teams through NCCDR. NCCDR serves as a resource for state or local child death review teams. NCCDR helps states share information by publishing their child death review teams' contact information, data, and annual reports on its Web site. In addition, NCCDR has developed a Web site designed to help child death review teams expand their prevention efforts. It offers best practices for preventing the leading causes of injury and death among children, including child abuse. The site contains links to resources, partners, and a number of injury prevention strategies including public education; legislation and policy changes; and modifications to products, physical environments, and social environments that have been rated according to their evidence-based effectiveness.

Although NCCDR regularly collaborates with federal organizations to analyze child fatality data and develop strategies to prevent child deaths, there has been little routine information sharing between NCCDR and NCANDS on child maltreatment fatalities. Federal organizations such as CDC, the Department of Defense, and the National Highway Traffic Safety Administration have collaborated with NCCDR to analyze information and expertise about child death reviews and develop prevention strategies, according to NCCDR officials. For example, in 2003, CDC developed an initiative to improve data collected on sudden unexplained infant deaths (SUID) and develop prevention strategies by monitoring trends and identifying risk factors. CDC partnered with NCCDR to develop the SUID Case Registry Pilot Study, which utilized an updated version of NCCDR's Web-based data collection system. Officials from NCCDR and the Children's Bureau, under HHS's Administration for Children and Families (ACF), meet periodically in workgroups, and officials from the Children's Bureau told us that they refer states with questions about child death reviews to NCCDR for assistance.[61] In 2010, officials from NCCDR and the ACF Commissioner met to explore ways to enhance federal responses to child abuse deaths, and the ACF Commissioner told us that they are moving forward to fund a child fatality review conference and begin an initiative to examine evidence-based practices for preventing child abuse deaths. However, NCCDR and NCANDS officials acknowledged that, to date, they have not routinely coordinated on child maltreatment fatality data or prevention strategies.

States Would Like Additional Assistance in Collecting and Using Data on Child Fatalities and Near Fatalities from Maltreatment

Although HHS provides a variety of assistance to states on how to report data to NCANDS, state officials indicated a need for additional assistance collecting child fatality as well as near-fatality data to use for prevention efforts.

Assistance Collecting Fatality Data

In our survey, almost half of states (23) reported needing additional assistance in collecting information and reporting data on child maltreatment fatalities or near fatalities. For example, several states mentioned that assistance with multidisciplinary coordination could help them overcome difficulties such as obtaining death certificates from medical examiners' or coroner's offices. HHS recognizes that collecting maltreatment fatality data from multiple sources results in more complete data, so the agency encourages states to coordinate with other organizations, such as medical examiners and departments of health. HHS officials stated that this is often a topic of discussion at the NCANDS annual meeting. However, HHS officials also noted that the agency cannot require states to use additional data sources, and states are not required to disclose whether they consulted with additional sources to collect data.

Collecting Maltreatment Data on Near Fatalities

Although the federal government does not currently collect data on children who nearly die from maltreatment, states reported wanting assistance to collect and use this information. CAPTA defines a near fatality as "an act that, as certified by a physician, places the child in serious or critical condition." HHS officials believe that such cases are most likely reported generally under maltreatment, but are not specifically identified as near fatalities because NCANDS does not have a data field identifying the case as a near fatality. HHS officials said it would be difficult to operationalize a national definition. To add a near-fatality data element to NCANDS, HHS would need to coordinate with the State Advisory Group and obtain approval from the Office of Management and Budget (OMB). However, the entire NCANDS data form will need to be reapproved in 2012, and HHS officials stated that at that time all NCANDS data elements will be reexamined.[62] In commenting on a draft of this report, HHS stated that it had initiated consultations with the states on how to best address data collection on near fatalities of children and that HHS is considering adding a field to identify these specific cases.

States are increasingly interested in collecting and using information on near fatalities, according to HHS officials, and some states have already begun this effort. Collecting data on maltreatment near fatalities was a topic of discussion at the 2010 NCANDS Annual State Technical Assistance Meeting. Additionally, the NCANDS Listserv was recently used by two state officials to survey other states about how they review and define near-fatality cases of maltreatment. Currently, states' definition of a near fatality varies (see figure 8), and to establish a near-fatality data element in NCANDS, states may need to reexamine their existing definitions. According to our survey results, 32 states have a state law, statute, or policy that defines a near fatality, and 19 states already collect data on the number of child near fatalities from maltreatment. In addition, some states obtain information on the circumstances

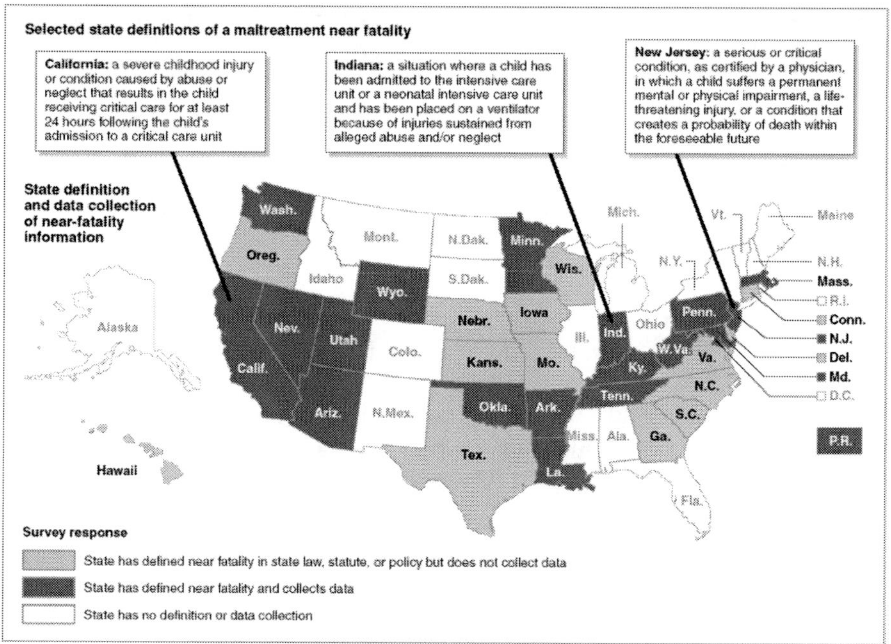

Source: GAO survey of states and state near-fatality definitions; MapInfo (map).

Note: State definitions may be included in a regulation or action by a state administrative agency. Calif. Dept. of Social Services, ACL No. 08-13 (March 14, 2008), p.1, fn.1; Indiana Dept. of Child Services, Child Welfare Manual, p.5 (Aug. 1, 2010); N.J. Admin. Code § 10:133-1.3 (2011).

Figure 8. State Variation in Defining and Collecting Information on Child Maltreatment Near Fatalities.

of child maltreatment near fatalities, such as the child's age and ethnicity, the child's relationship to the perpetrator, and whether the child was receiving foster care or family preservation services.

Assistance on Using Data for Prevention

States predominantly use child maltreatment fatality and near-fatality data to develop strategies for preventing these occurrences, and state officials told us they would like more assistance to use this information for prevention. States reported in our survey that child maltreatment fatality data are often used to inform prevention strategies, make state-level child welfare policy changes, and allocate funding or other resources for prevention activities. In addition, states reported using the information they collect on child maltreatment near fatalities to inform or implement strategies for preventing maltreatment fatalities and to allocate funding or other resources for prevention activities. For example, as a result of trends associated with fatal maltreatment and crying infants, many states have developed public awareness campaigns, resources for parents, and other interventions to prevent shaken baby syndrome (see sidebar).

STATE SHAKEN BABY CAMPAIGNS

Shaken baby syndrome, which is associated with the violent shaking of an infant or young child, usually occurs when a caretaker becomes frustrated with a crying child. Prevention efforts typically include educating new parents on the dangers of shaken baby syndrome and offering coping mechanisms to resolve parental anger or frustration. Many states, including California, New York, and Wisconsin, currently have prevention campaigns that specifically target new parents at hospitals, places of birth, or other health care facilities. Ten states have statewide public awareness campaigns, and two states have passed legislation to include education in public schools on parental skills and responsibility, including the dangers of shaking infants, according to the National Conference of State Legislatures.

Source: GAO analysis of information from NCSL.

HHS officials confirmed that states were increasingly interested in receiving technical assistance on how to use child fatality data to meaningfully inform prevention efforts. State officials also reported wanting more information from other states on best practices in general and on using data for prevention efforts in particular.

CONCLUSION

In conclusion, children's deaths from maltreatment are especially distressing because they involve a failure on the part of adults responsible for protecting them. Child welfare policymakers and practitioners rely on child maltreatment fatality data—voluntarily reported by states—to understand the extent and circumstances of these tragic deaths and to develop strategies to prevent them. At the state level, obtaining comprehensive data on child maltreatment fatalities is very challenging and requires information sharing among state and local agencies—each with its own policies, types and levels of expertise, and concerns. Yet such cooperative efforts are a work in progress, and assistance from HHS to help states collect and report more comprehensive child fatality data is important. At the federal level, to the extent that HHS collects but does not publish information on child maltreatment fatalities, or does not routinely share information on child fatality data analyses, opportunities may be lost to identify effective means of preventing child maltreatment deaths in the future. Finally, without national data on children's near fatalities from maltreatment, we are unable to have a clear picture of the extent of near fatalities and the risk factors associated with such maltreatment, making it difficult to develop prevention strategies. As a society, we should be doing everything in our collective power to end child deaths and near deaths from maltreatment, and the collection and reporting of comprehensive data on these tragic situations is an important step toward that goal.

RECOMMENDATIONS FOR EXECUTIVE ACTION

To improve the comprehensiveness, quality, and use of national data on child fatalities from maltreatment, the Secretary of HHS should take the following four actions

1. Identify ways to help states strengthen the completeness and reliability of data they report to NCANDS. These efforts could include identifying and sharing states' best practices, particularly those that foster cross-agency coordination and help address differences in state definitions and interpretation of maltreatment and/or privacy and confidentiality concerns.
2. Expand, as appropriate, the type and amount of information HHS makes public on the circumstances surrounding child fatalities from maltreatment.
3. Use stronger mechanisms to routinely share analyses and expertise with its partners on the circumstances of child maltreatment deaths, including insights that could be used for developing prevention strategies.

4. Estimate the costs and benefits of collecting national data on near fatalities and take appropriate follow-up actions.

AGENCY COMMENTS AND OUR EVALUATION

We provided a draft of this report to HHS for review and comment, and HHS's comments are reproduced in appendix IV. We also provided a draft of this report to the Department of Justice (DOJ) and pertinent excerpts to NCCDR. DOJ and NCCDR provided technical comments, which we incorporated as appropriate.

In its comments, HHS agreed with our recommendations to improve the comprehensiveness, quality, and use of national data on child fatalities from maltreatment. HHS also provided technical comments and additional information about activities under way or planned, which we incorporated as appropriate. For example, HHS stated that it has initiated conversations with the states to improve the identification of cases that involve near fatalities and that it plans to include two additional analyses on child fatalities in the Child Maltreatment report in 2013. While we recognize that HHS has some activities under way pertinent to issues raised in our report, more can be done to address these issues, such as by using stronger mechanisms to routinely share information and expertise on child fatalities from maltreatment. For example, although HHS cites the Federal Inter-agency Work Group on Child Abuse and Neglect as a mechanism already in place for sharing information, HHS officials previously told us that this workgroup has not often discussed child fatalities from maltreatment. Since having mechanisms is a starting point for information sharing, we clarified our recommendation to emphasize the importance of putting such means to routine use. HHS also noted that NCANDS data collection has always been voluntary, as our report acknowledges.

In its comments, HHS also raised concerns about the nationwide Web-based survey of child welfare administrators—one of several methodologies used for this report—noting that it had several limitations. According to HHS, survey completion was typically delegated to subordinates, which can create inconsistencies in the types of respondents and data collected; the staff person responding may not have considered information from other divisions; and finally, states provided self-reported information and thus GAO cannot validate it. For the most part, these observations would apply to any survey in which the respondent is answering the survey questions as a representative of an organization rather than as an individual. We took several precautions to minimize these limitations. For example, before activating the survey, we confirmed that the state officials listed were correct for completing the survey; obtained comments on the survey draft from three experts, in addition to conducting pretests with state officials; and provided respondents ample time for consultation with other state officials as needed. We received responses from all states. While survey data are not typically verified independently, in our judgment the precautions taken to address survey limitations are sufficient for our purposes. (App. I provides information on our survey methodology.).

Sincerely yours,

Kay E. Brown
Director, Education, Workforce, and Income Security Issues

APPENDIX I. SCOPE AND METHODOLOGY

Survey of States

To obtain state perspectives on our objectives, we conducted a Web-based survey of child welfare administrators in the 50 states, the District of Columbia, and Puerto Rico. The survey was conducted using a self-administered electronic questionnaire posted on the Web. HHS provided us with names and contact information for state child welfare administrators. We contacted child welfare administrators via e-mail announcing the survey and sent follow-up e-mails to encourage responses. The survey data were collected between October and December 2010, with child welfare officials from every state, the District of Columbia, and Puerto Rico responding. The survey included questions about state laws related to child maltreatment, child welfare department coordination with other agencies or entities, state challenges related to identifying and collecting information on child maltreatment fatalities and reporting these data to NCANDS, child death review teams, state challenges related to collecting information on child maltreatment near fatalities, and federal assistance from HHS to states on data collection and reporting.

We worked with agency officials and experts to develop the survey. Because this was not a sample survey, there are no sampling errors. However, the practical difficulties of conducting any survey may introduce errors, commonly referred to as nonsampling errors. For example, differences in how a particular question is interpreted or in the sources of information that are available to respondents can introduce unwanted variability into the survey results. We took steps in the development of the survey, data collection, and data analysis to minimize these nonsampling errors. For example, prior to administering the survey, we pretested the content and format of the survey with four states (Arizona, Kansas, New York, and Wisconsin) to determine whether (1) the survey questions were clear, (2) the terms used were precise and accurate, (3) respondents were able to provide the information we were seeking, and (4) the questions were unbiased. We chose these pretest states based on a number of factors, including recommendations from HHS officials or experts, whether the state collected information on near fatalities from maltreatment, whether the state had a state-level child death review team, and overall child population, among others. We made changes to the content and format of the final survey based on pretest results. Because this was a Web-based survey in which respondents entered their responses directly into our database, there was a reduced possibility of data entry error. We also performed computer analyses to identify inconsistencies in responses and other indications of error. In addition, an independent analyst verified that the computer programs used to analyze these data were written correctly.

Literature Review

To identify research that estimated the number of child deaths from maltreatment in the United States and the extent to which these deaths are accurately captured, or undercounted, we searched ProQuest, Dialog Social Science Databases, NTIS, SocAbs, Nexis Statistical Master File, and MEDLINE. We also asked researchers and subject matter experts to identify studies. We selected 19 studies that had been published after 2000; had a focus on the child fatality data collection process in the United States; had a state or national, rather than county-level, focus; and focused on child maltreatment fatalities, not abuse and neglect. For each selected study, we determined whether the study's findings were generally reliable. Two GAO social science analysts assessed each study's research methodology, including its research design, sampling frame, selection of measure, data quality, limitation, and analytic techniques for its methodological soundness and the validity of the results and conclusions that were drawn.

NCANDS Data Analysis

To identify the extent to which HHS collects and provides comprehensive information on child fatalities from maltreatment, we obtained and analyzed NCANDS data from the National Data Archive on Child Abuse and Neglect (NDACAN) at Cornell University. NDACAN prepares data and documentation for secondary analysis, and disseminates the datasets to researchers. We obtained the NCANDS datasets for federal fiscal year 2009 from NDACAN for our analysis. The NCANDS datasets consist of files in three formats: the child file, the agency file, and the summary data component (SDC). The child file dataset is the case-level component of NCANDS that contains child-specific data of all state CPS investigations or assessments of alleged child maltreatment that received a disposition during fiscal year 2009. Fifty states submitted the child file in fiscal year 2009, including the District of Columbia and Puerto Rico. The agency file is the NCANDS state-level component, which is submitted by states that submit the child file. The agency file contains aggregated state-level data that have been requested by CAPTA that are not able to be collected at the case level. This includes data on preventative services, CPS workload, and child fatalities not reported at the case level in the child file. For fiscal year 2009, 50 states submitted the agency file. States that are unable to submit case-level data submit the SDC file. The SDC consists of aggregated state-level statistics of key items in the child file and agency file. (Two states submitted the SDC for fiscal year 2009.)

Both states and NDACAN take steps to protect confidentiality. States encrypt all identification variables submitted to NCANDS to prevent tracing a child file record back to the record in the state's child welfare information system. For records involving a fatality, NDACAN recodes certain variables to mask information, including the state, county of report, information about the child, and perpetrator identification.

We analyzed a subset of fiscal year 2009 NCANDS child file cases in which a child maltreatment fatality had occurred (i.e., those in which the maltreatment death data element was equal to 1 or "yes"). Data elements that were analyzed included age, sex, maltreatment type, and perpetrator characteristics. In addition to the analysis of fiscal year 2009 child file cases in which a maltreatment death had occurred, we analyzed four variables each from the fiscal year 2009 agency file and SDC. These four variables were the number of child maltreatment fatalities, foster care deaths, children whose families had received family preservation services in the 5 years prior to fiscal year 2009, and children who had been in foster care and were reunited with their families in the 5 years prior to fiscal year 2009. These agency file and SDC variables were summed with the equivalent child file variables to yield complete totals.

We assessed the reliability of the NCANDS data provided by NDACAN by conducting electronic testing; reviewing documentation on the NCANDS data; and interviewing officials from NDACAN, the NCANDS contractor (Walter R. McDonald & Associates), and the Children's Bureau of HHS to clarify data elements and procedures for data collection and reporting. To verify the number of unduplicated fatalities due to child maltreatment, we compared our assessment with the analysis done by NDACAN researchers. The NCANDS data were found to be sufficiently reliable for the purposes of this engagement.

NCCDR Data Analysis

To examine the extent to which HHS collects and provides comprehensive information on child fatalities from maltreatment, we requested and obtained state child death review team data from NCCDR's Child Death Review (CDR) Case Reporting System. The CDR Case Reporting System is a Web-based application that allows local and state users to enter case data and access and download their data via the Internet on a continual and voluntary basis. In 2009, state and local child death review teams in 26 states submitted data to the CDR Case Reporting System. These data contain detailed information on the child welfare history of victims, including the number of CPS referrals and substantiations per child, whether there was an open CPS case at the time of death, and whether any siblings were ever put in foster care. The database contains extensive information on the incident that led to the death, including the place of the incident, such as the child's home, and the type of injury that caused the death, such as a weapon or drowning. The system also collects information on acts of commission or omission for every death entered into the system, regardless of cause or manner. To confirm the reliability of these data, social science methodologists at GAO reviewed documentation about the collection and reporting of NCCDR data. We also interviewed several NCCDR officials who were responsible for these data and HHS officials responsible for the cooperative agreement with NCCDR. In addition, we compared NCCDR data on child fatalities with NCANDS data on child fatalities in the NCCDR states. Although these data were not sufficiently reliable to support a finding, they were reliable for providing background context and examples of the possible data elements not available from NCANDS.

Site Visits

To gather additional information about challenges states face in collecting and reporting information on child maltreatment fatalities to NCANDS, including challenges at the local level, and federal assistance to states, we conducted site visits to California, Michigan, and Pennsylvania and met with state officials and officials from selected localities within those states between July and December 2010. Specifically, we met with local officials from Calaveras, Los Angeles, and Sacramento counties in California; Bay, Genessee, Ingham, Lincoln, Oakland, and Wayne counties in Michigan; and Berks, Lehigh, and Philadelphia counties, among others, in Pennsylvania.[63]

We selected these states based on recommendations from HHS officials and experts, child population, collection of information on child maltreatment near fatalities, type of child welfare program administration (state-administered and county-administered with state supervision), and geographic diversity. We worked with state officials to select counties that were located in both urban and rural areas to ensure that we captured any related differences in data collection and reporting processes and federal assistance. During these visits, we interviewed state child welfare officials and officials from the department of health or other body coordinating the child death review process, and collected relevant state laws, policies, procedures, and reports. At the local level, we interviewed CPS officials, law enforcement personnel, and medical examiners or coroners in charge of investigating child deaths in each state. Through these interviews, we collected information on state and local processes for collecting and reporting data on child maltreatment fatalities and the associated challenges officials face. We conducted some of these interviews via telephone to limit travel costs.

Information we gathered on our site visits represents only the conditions present in the states and local areas at the time of our site visits. We cannot comment on any changes that may have occurred after our fieldwork was completed. Furthermore, our fieldwork focused on in-depth analysis of only a few selected states. On the basis of our site visit information, we cannot generalize our findings beyond the states we visited.

Expert Interviews

For all three objectives, we interviewed HHS officials and other experts on child maltreatment fatalities and near fatalities. We identified child maltreatment researchers through our literature review and through recommendations from stakeholders knowledgeable about child maltreatment fatalities and near fatalities. For this study, we interviewed HHS and other officials knowledgeable about NCANDS, NCCDR, and NIS-4 data. We also interviewed researchers and experts affiliated with the following centers and associations: the American Academy of Pediatrics (AAP), the American Bar Association's (ABA) Center on Children and the Law, the Child Welfare League of America, the National Coalition to End Child Abuse Deaths, the Interagency Council for Child Abuse and Neglect/National Center on Child Fatality Review, and NCCDR. (The National Coalition to End Child Abuse Deaths includes officials from the Every Child Matters Education Fund, the National Center for Child Death Review, the National District Attorneys Association/National Center for Prosecution of Child Abuse, the National Association of Social Workers, and the National Children's Alliance.)

We conducted this performance audit from April 2010 through July 2011 in accordance with generally accepted government auditing standards. These standards require that we plan and perform the audit to obtain sufficient, appropriate evidence to provide a reasonable basis for our findings and conclusions based on our audit objectives. We believe that the evidence obtained provides a reasonable basis for our findings and conclusions based on our audit objectives.

APPENDIX II. SELECTED INFORMATION ON CHILD FATALITIES FROM MALTREATMENT

Table 3. Information Collected by NCANDS on Child Maltreatment Fatalities

Type of child maltreatment data collected by NCANDS	Selected NCANDS results on child fatalities from maltreatment reported by HHS for fiscal year 2009
Information about the child	• Forty-six percent of fatalities were children younger than 1 year, and 81 percent were 3 years old or younger. • Boys had a slightly higher child fatality rate than girls, at 2.36 per 100,000 boys in the population, and girls had a

Type of child maltreatment data collected by NCANDS	Selected NCANDS results on child fatalities from maltreatment reported by HHS for fiscal year 2009
	rate of 2.12 per 100,000 girls in the population. • Of all child fatalities, 39 percent were White children, 29 percent were African-American, and 17 percent were Hispanic. Children of American Indian or Alaska Native, Asian, Pacific Islander, or multiple race categories collectively accounted for 3.6 percent, and 11.2 percent were children of unknown race.
Type(s) of maltreatment[a]	• Thirty-seven percent of child fatalities were caused by multiple forms of maltreatment. • Neglect accounted for about 36 percent of fatalities and physical abuse for 23 percent.
Information about perpetrators[b]	• Seventy-six percent of child fatalities were caused by one or more parents. • Twenty-seven percent of child fatalities were perpetrated by the mother acting alone, and 23 percent were caused by both parents. • Foster parents and legal guardians accounted for less than 1 percent of perpetrators (foster parents were reported as the perpetrator in 5 child fatalities from maltreatment).
Child welfare contact	• Twelve percent of children who died from maltreatment were from families who had received family preservation services in the previous 5 years.[c] • Two percent of children who died from maltreatment had been in foster care and were reunited with their families in the previous 5 years.[d]
Child's risk factors[e] Risk factors associated with the caregiver[f] Preventive services provided to families[g]	• HHS's *Child Maltreatment 2009* report did not provide information on these data elements for children who died from maltreatment.

Source: HHS, Child Maltreatment 2009.

Notes: States report these data on a child-specific level through NCANDS child files.

[a] Maltreatment types include neglect, physical abuse, sexual abuse, psychological maltreatment, and medical neglect.

[b] NCANDS defines a perpetrator as a person determined to have caused or knowingly allowed the maltreatment of a child.

[c] Family preservation services are activities designed to help families alleviate crises that might lead to out-of-home placement of children, maintain the safety of children in their own homes, support families preparing to reunify or adopt, and assist families in obtaining services and other supports necessary to address their multiple needs.

[d] This information is provided through aggregated agency files rather than individual case-level child files. Data are for fiscal year 2009. HHS also collects data on children who died from maltreatment while in foster care. However, the foster care data element is ambiguous because child deaths while in foster care can

reflect earlier maltreatment by parents that led to the child's removal from the home, deaths from other causes such as disease or accidents, or deaths from maltreatment by foster parents. Perpetrator information is more useful: In fiscal year 2009, foster parents were reported as the perpetrator in 5 child fatalities from maltreatment.

[e] Child risk factors include having an intellectual disability, physical disability, learning disability, and visual or hearing impairment.

[f] Risk factors associated with the caregiver include alcohol or drug abuse, domestic violence, emotional disturbance, and financial difficulties.

[g] Preventive services are provided to parents whose children are at risk of maltreatment and include family support, child day care, education and training, employment, and housing.

Information from NCCDR on Child Maltreatment Fatalities

Following are selected results from our analysis of child maltreatment data in the CDR Reporting System:[64]

Manner of death: Homicide was the manner of death on the death certificate for 57 percent of child maltreatment fatality victims reported to NCCDR in calendar year 2009.

Cause of death: Injury was the primary cause of death for 79 percent of children who died from maltreatment, and just over half of those children were killed with a weapon.

Child welfare history: Of the 417 reported child maltreatment fatality victims:

- Thirty-one percent had a documented history of maltreatment.[65]
- Thirteen percent had an open CPS case prior to the incident causing the child's death.
- Fourteen percent of children who died had at least one CPS referral prior to their deaths.
- Eight percent were placed in foster care prior to their deaths.[66]

Appendix III. Information from States Not Reported in NCANDS

State Data on Child Fatalities Not Reported to NCANDS

Thirty-two states also collected information on child maltreatment fatalities that were not reported to NCANDS in fiscal year 2009, according to our survey of state child welfare officials. For example, 27 states reported that they collected data on the child's family characteristics that they did not report to NCANDS in fiscal year 2009. (See table 4.) Data that states collect but do not report to NCANDS could represent additional, more detailed information on children who die from maltreatment (such as information on siblings' prior contact with the child welfare system) or data that states collect but cannot report for technical reasons. For example, in explaining this condition, two states noted that much of the data was captured in narrative or case logs—not in reportable data fields—while another state noted that it collects additional information on child maltreatment fatalities reported by local county child welfare agencies.

Table 4. Types of Child Fatality Data States Collected but Did Not Report to NCANDS

Types of child fatality data elements not reported to NCANDS in fiscal year 2009	Number of states collecting data
Child information (e.g., maltreatment history, mental health, criminal history)	29
Child's status in relation to the child welfare system (e.g., foster care or prior substantiated maltreatment)	29
Incident information (e.g., date, time, place)	28
Primary cause of death	27
Family characteristics (e.g., sibling information, siblings' prior contact with child welfare system)	27
Information about person responsible for supervising child at time of near death if the supervisor was not the primary caregiver (e.g., demographic, criminal history)	26
Information about child's primary caregiver (e.g., employment, education level, criminal history)	25

Source: GAO survey of state child welfare officials.

APPENDIX IV. COMMENTS FROM THE DEPARTMENT OF HEALTH AND HUMAN SERVICES

DEPARTMENT OF HEALTH & HUMAN SERVICES

OFFICE OF THE SECRETARY

Assistant Secretary for Legislation
Washington, DC 20201

JUN 20 2011

Kay Brown
Director, Education, Workforce
and Income Security Issues
U.S. Government Accountability Office
441 G Street N.W.
Washington, DC 20548

Dear Ms. Brown:

Attached are comments on the U.S. Government Accountability Office's (GAO) draft report entitled, "CHILD MALTREATMENT: Strengthening National Data on Child Fatalities Could Aid in Prevention" (GAO 11-599).

The Department appreciates the opportunity to review this report prior to publication.

Sincerely,

Jim R. Esquea
Assistant Secretary for Legislation

Attachment

GENERAL COMMENTS OF THE DEPARTMENT OF HEALTH AND HUMAN SERVICES (HHS) ON THE GOVERNMENT ACCOUNTABILITY OFFICE'S (GAO) DRAFT REPORT ENTITLED, "CHILD MALTREATMENT: STRENGTHENING NATIONAL DATA ON CHILD FATALITIES COULD AID IN PREVENTION" (GAO-11-599)

The Department appreciates the opportunity to review and comment on this draft report.

GAO Recommendations

To improve the comprehensiveness, quality, and use of national data on child fatalities from maltreatment, the Secretary of HHS should:

1. Identify ways to help States strengthen the completeness and reliability of data they report to NCANDS. These efforts could include identifying and sharing states best practices, particularly those that foster cross-agency coordination and help address differences in state definitions and interpretation of maltreatment and/or privacy and confidentiality concerns.
2. Expand, as appropriate, the type and amount of information HHS makes public on the circumstances surrounding child fatalities from maltreatment.
3. Establish routine mechanisms for HHS agencies and their partners to share analyses and expertise on the circumstances of child maltreatment deaths, including insights that could be used for developing prevention strategies.
4. Estimate the costs and benefits of collecting national data on near fatalities and take appropriate follow up actions.

Administration for Children and Families (ACF) Response

GAO's recommendations essentially suggest ACF's Administration on Children, Youth and Families (ACYF) continue activities currently under way and activities that will continue into the future. ACYF is in agreement with the GAO recommendations and the comments below elaborate on the work already under way or planned.

Several processes and forums are in place for furthering these dialogues. The Children's Bureau (CB) continues to provide detailed annual reports on child maltreatment that identify and address interpretation issues. Thus readers can use the information to conduct their own research or form their own interpretations.

The annual publication of Child Maltreatment is updated and expanded each year. The full data file is available from the National Data Archive on Child Abuse. There are approximately 56 tables planned for the *Child Maltreatment 2010* report, compared to 51 tables in the 2009 report. Two additional tables on fatalities have been planned for some time and will be included in the

GENERAL COMMENTS OF THE DEPARTMENT OF HEALTH AND HUMAN SERVICES (HHS) ON THE GOVERNMENT ACCOUNTABILITY OFFICE'S (GAO) DRAFT REPORT ENTITLED, "CHILD MALTREATMENT: STRENGTHENING NATIONAL DATA ON CHILD FATALITIES COULD AID IN PREVENTION" (GAO-11-599)

report. The full data file is available from the National Data Archive on Child Abuse and Neglect at Cornell University for researchers to use after the annual report is released.

Two relevant issues are: 1) CB does not have statutory authority to require States to provide this data; it has always been a voluntary effort and, under the Child Abuse Prevention and Treatment Act (CAPTA), "to the extent practicable," and 2) the data reported is meant to be nationally representative, that is, reflective of what is happening in all of the States. Some data elements are not discussed at length in the report when there is not sufficient input from the States.

Several mechanisms are already in place for sharing of information. The Federal Inter-Agency Work Group on Child Abuse and Neglect serves as a coordinating group. CB manages the Children's Justice Act (CJA) under CAPTA. One of the key tenets of CJA is that funds be spent on improving the handling of abuse-related fatalities. Many of the States have used their funding over the years to establish and support local and State child fatality review teams, which include a data collection component. CB hosts the CJA grantees meeting as well as the State Liaison meeting annually, and the National Child Abuse and Neglect Data System (NCANDS) data team members participate in those meetings. The 18th National Conference on Child Abuse and Neglect will be hosted by CB in April 2012. At this Conference, as well as in many previous years of the Conference, opportunities exist for workshops, roundtable discussions, exhibit area and poster session interaction on these topics. Finally, the CB enjoys a positive working relationship with the Health Resources and Services Administration (HRSA) and the National Center for Child Death Review (NCCDR), which it funds.

CB has already initiated conversations with the States to improve the identification of cases that involve near fatalities. With the support of the States, it is anticipated that the Child File of NCANDS will be modified to include an additional data element identifying such cases.

National Child Abuse and Neglect Data System

The national data reported to the Department via NCANDS is the most comprehensive data on child maltreatment that our Nation has ever had. This is also true for the data on child fatalities. For 2009, case-level data for more than 3.5 million records of child abuse and neglect were reported and analyzed by HHS. This includes case-level data for more than 1,300 fatalities. We consider this a major achievement given the following factors:

- Participation by the States in NCANDS is voluntary. The combined effort of the States and CB results in an annual report each year.
- States do not receive additional funding for participation in NCANDS, and yet contribute staff time each year, as their resources allow.
- Definitions of child abuse and neglect and procedures for responding to allegations of maltreatment are established by state legislative and departmental authority.

GENERAL COMMENTS OF THE DEPARTMENT OF HEALTH AND HUMAN SERVICES (HHS) ON THE GOVERNMENT ACCOUNTABILITY OFFICE'S (GAO) DRAFT REPORT ENTITLED, "CHILD MALTREATMENT: STRENGTHENING NATIONAL DATA ON CHILD FATALITIES COULD AID IN PREVENTION" (GAO-11-599)

- Reporting of child maltreatment and child fatalities is the responsibility of the public by both professional and community members. Each year, more than 1 million professionals undertake the responsibility for reporting alleged abuse and neglect.

CB routinely coordinates the reporting of improved data to NCANDS with the efforts of States to develop and improve their information system through the Division of State Systems; to respond to Federally mandated state reporting requirements for foster care and independent living through the Division of Program Implementation; to receive a wide range of technical assistance through 10 national resource centers overseen by the Division of Child Welfare Capacity; and to receive grant funding for prevention activities. Additionally, CB has created a number of quality improvement centers to further innovation in child protective services throughout the United States. The Office of Child Abuse and Neglect serves as the link between the CB and other initiatives, which address child maltreatment.

While it is commonly believed that the reported number of children who were known to have died due to child abuse and neglect is an undercount, we are making considerable progress in closing the gap between deaths due to child maltreatment and those that are not identified as such. HHS supports States in their use of primary prevention to help parents be more aware of the dangers of co-sleeping; unsecured weapons and medications; and unsupervised play. The 18th National Conference on Child Abuse and Neglect in 2012, which is likely to draw more than 2,000 attendees, will include several sessions related to preventing and addressing child fatalities and near fatalities. Additionally, the annual Child Maltreatment report in 2013 will have two additional analyses in the chapter about child fatalities. The additional analyses will examine caregiver risk factors of children who died and the total number of reported fatalities by state during the previous five years.

Adding new data elements for the States to report as part of the NCANDS data file is undertaken in a systematic manner. All potential new data fields are discussed with the States for the feasibility of collecting and reporting the data via NCANDS. Each potential new data field must go through the Office of Management and Budget review and approval cycle before it can be implemented as a reportable field in the NCANDS data file. Consultations with the States have already been initiated to determine how to best address data collection on near fatalities of children. The feasibility of collecting and reporting data on Shaken Baby Syndrome (also known as inflicted traumatic brain injury) will be discussed with States this summer.

National Resource Center on Child Protective Services

It is important to clarify the current involvement of the National Resource Center (NRC) on Child Protective Services (CPS). NRC has on occasion received requests for technical assistance on improving a State's child fatality review system, and has responded to those requests. In addition, there is one consultant at NRC specifically designated to respond to queries from Citizen Review Panels. NRC has a good working relationship with the National Center on Child

GENERAL COMMENTS OF THE DEPARTMENT OF HEALTH AND HUMAN SERVICES (HHS) ON THE GOVERNMENT ACCOUNTABILITY OFFICE'S (GAO) DRAFT REPORT ENTITLED, "CHILD MALTREATMENT: STRENGTHENING NATIONAL DATA ON CHILD FATALITIES COULD AID IN PREVENTION" (GAO-11-599)

Death Review and often refers constituents to the Center. Additionally, NRC is often called in to help States after a child fatality has occurred, to review their CPS system and determine if the fatality could have been prevented. In a recent example, one State has decided to redesign its system, particularly in the area of safety decision making, which is a critical first step in the CPS response process.

Limitations of the GAO Review

GAO conducted a nationwide web-based survey of State child welfare administrators as part of their data collection and analysis to complete the report and provide recommendations. This type of data collection and analysis has methodological limitations to include: 1) In many States, Commissioners/Directors do not complete the survey. Completion of the survey is typically delegated to subordinates, which results in 50 States selecting different staff at different levels of experience, with different backgrounds and from different divisions to complete the survey. This creates inconsistencies in respondents and the data collected. 2) The staff person responding to the survey may not have considered input from various divisions such as the IT division, Critical Review/Child Death Unit, etc. Some agencies have both an internal review unit and a statewide multidisciplinary review unit and including both perspectives would be critical. 3) The survey data collected is self-report, with no ability for the GAO to validate information provided.

End Notes

[1] In this report, we use the term "maltreatment" to refer to both abuse and neglect, unless noted otherwise, which is also consistent with the Department of Health and Human Service's use of the term in its annual report, *Child Maltreatment*.

[2] In this report, we use the terms "child fatalities" and "child deaths" interchangeably.

[3] Child Abuse Prevention, Adoption, and Family Services Act of 1988, Pub. L. No. 100-294, sec. 101, § 6(b)(1), 102 Stat. 102, 107.

[4] Throughout this report, references to state survey responses include the District of Columbia and Puerto Rico.

[5] We selected our site visit states based on expert recommendations and variations in demographics, child welfare program administrative structure, and other factors. During these site visits, we interviewed state child welfare officials and state child death review team officials, as well as county or local officials from child protective services, law enforcement, coroner or medical examiner offices, and others involved in child death investigations or review processes.

[6] CDC's National Center for Health Statistics (NCHS) collects information from death certificates. This figure includes deaths of children from birth to age 19.

[7] The perinatal period refers to the weeks immediately before and after birth; a congenital anomaly is a health problem or a physical abnormality that a baby has at birth.

[8] Fiscal year 2009 data are the most recent information on child maltreatment from NCANDS. With regard to child fatalities, 49 states reported a total of 1,676 child fatalities from maltreatment to HHS. Of those 49 states, 44 reported child-specific, case-level data on 1,343 fatalities, and 40 reported aggregate data on an additional 333 fatalities. On the basis of these data, HHS estimates that 1,770 children died from maltreatment in fiscal year 2009.

Alaska, Massachusetts, and North Carolina did not report data on child fatalities for fiscal year 2009.

[9] In the majority of states, child welfare programs are state administered through state and local offices, while in a minority of states, they are state supervised and county administered, according to HHS.

[10] After investigation or assessment, the allegations are either "substantiated" or "founded" or "unsubstantiated/ unfounded," according to HHS. In some states, CPS focuses on the service needs of the family if the child is considered at low or medium risk of harm rather than investigating allegations of maltreatment. This approach is called "alternative response" or "differential response."

[11] In the case of child deaths in which there has been no previous contact with child welfare services, law enforcement officials and medical examiners or coroners may conduct investigations without CPS. The results of these investigations may or may not be reported to CPS agencies.

[12] HHS's Children's Bureau in the Administration for Children and Families (ACF) sponsors 10 NRCs that provide individualized training and technical assistance to states and localities, by request, on various topics.

[13] 42 U.S.C. §§ 5104, 5105. CAPTA Reauthorization Act of 2010, Pub. L. No. 111-320, 124 Stat. 3459.

[14] Under this grant, each eligible state receives a base allotment of $50,000. Remaining funds are distributed in proportion to each state's relative share of the child population under 18 among all states that apply for a grant. 42 U.S.C. § 5106a(f)(2). CAPTA funding is included in the $8.4 billion in federal funds provided for child welfare programs in fiscal year 2010.

[15] 42 U.S.C. § 5106a(b)(1), (2), and § 5106g(2).

[16] See 42 U.S.C. § 5106a(c).

[17] CAPTA also defines "serious bodily injury" as "bodily injury which involves substantial risk of death, extreme physical pain, protracted and obvious disfigurement, or protracted loss or impairment of the function of a bodily member, organ, or mental faculty." 42 U.S.C.§ 5106a(b)(4)(A), (B).

[18] Citizen review panels are authorized to review near fatalities. 42 U.S.C. § 5106a(c)(4)(A)(iii)(II).

[19] 42 U.S.C. § 5106a(d). Three CAPTA data items refer to child fatalities from maltreatment.

[20] Under CFSRs, established in 2000, states are assessed for substantial conformity with certain federal requirements for child protection, foster care, adoption, family preservation and family support, and independent living services. The CFSRs enable the Children's Bureau to (1) ensure conformity with federal child welfare requirements, (2) determine what is actually happening to children and families as they are engaged in child welfare services, and (3) assist states with enhancing their capacity to help children and families achieve positive outcomes.

[21] There is no separate file for child fatalities in NCANDS. A child's fatality is recorded as a data element in a child's individual case-level file that is maintained by state child welfare departments. State CPS agencies generally report data to NCANDS.

[22] NCANDS collects information on all children who were referred or reported to CPS because of alleged maltreatment and whose maltreatment was investigated or otherwise assessed. Such information is largely reported through individual case-level "child files." States that are unable to provide case-level data provide aggregated counts of key indicators through "agency files." As we note, states are also encouraged to go beyond CPS data in reporting child fatalities to NCANDS.

[23] In addition, some states do not report data on child maltreatment for residential treatment facilities to NCANDS, as we noted in our earlier work. Residential treatment facilities are boarding schools, academies, boot camps, and wilderness camps that provide services for children with behavioral or emotional challenges. Because many states lack authority under state law to gather data from some residential treatment facilities, such as exclusively

private facilities, we found that NCANDS data may understate the number of fatalities and other kinds of maltreatment occurring in such facilities. GAO recommended that HHS determine the barriers for states that do not report case-file data for residential facilities to NCANDS and explore options to help states address existing barriers. GAO, *Residential Facilities: State and Federal Oversight Gaps May Increase Risk to Youth Well-Being,* GAO-08-696T, (Washington, D.C.: Apr. 24, 2008), and *Residential Facilities: Improved Data and Enhanced Oversight Would Help Safeguard the Well-Being of Youth with Behavioral and Emotional Challenges,* GAO-08-346 (Washington, D.C.: May 13, 2008).

[24] Nearly all states and some counties have a "child death review team" comprising CPS workers, prosecutors, law enforcement, coroners or medical examiners, public health care providers, and others. These multidisciplinary teams review cases of child deaths for the purpose of follow-up and prevention.

[25] According to HHS officials, agency files were established in part to enable states to report information about child maltreatment obtained from non-CPS agencies that also investigate child maltreatment, such as state health and justice departments and, in the case of fatalities, medical examiners' offices. Agency files also contain information on funding sources for preventive services; information on referrals and reports to CPS, including CPS staffing; and contacts with court representatives. Child-specific case-level details are not available for fatality data gathered from external departments that are reported in the agency file. In fiscal year 2009, all but two states submitted agency files.

[26] This response reflects the number of states (24) that responded "no" to questions about whether they used any non-CPS data sources in reporting NCANDS data, using agency files. According to HHS, 40 states reported data to NCANDS in their agency files on child maltreatment fatalities that HHS officials believe were obtained from non-CPS agencies. (See table 4-1 in HHS, *Child Maltreatment 2009*.) Sixteen of these 40 states reported zero child fatalities in the agency file for fiscal year 2009, and HHS officials said these agencies consulted with external agencies to determine the zero count. However, our survey question specifically asked state child welfare officials whether their state's NCANDS agency file for fiscal year 2009 includes information on child maltreatment fatalities from specific state agencies or entities, and 24 states responded "no" to all agencies or entities. States responded similarly as to whether they used any non-CPS data sources in reporting NCANDS data using child files (23 responded "no"). HHS officials acknowledged that gathering information on child maltreatment fatalities from multiple sources needs attention.

[27] See app. I for a description of the scope and methodology for this study, including information about our review of relevant literature.

[28] P. G. Schnitzer et al, "Public Health Surveillance of Fatal Child Maltreatment: Analysis of 3 State Programs," *American Journal of Public Health*, February 2008, Vol. 98, No. 2.

[29] The small number of fatalities in the sample size limits the reliability of the NIS estimate for child fatalities from maltreatment. Because the sample size is small, the estimate has a large standard error. Taking this variance into account, the 95 percent confidence interval around the incidence of child maltreatment fatalities estimated by the NIS-4 indicates that the number of children who died from maltreatment in 2005-2006 is likely between 1,541 and 3,318.

[30] The next report is due no later than Dec. 20, 2014. 42 U.S.C. § 5105(a)(3).

[31] The NIS applies two definitional standards: the Harm Standard and the Endangerment Standard. The Harm Standard generally requires that an act or omission result in demonstrable harm in order to be classified as abuse or neglect. (The incidence of child fatalities was reported under the Harm Standard.) The Endangerment Standard includes all children who meet the Harm Standard but adds children who were not yet harmed by abuse or neglect if a trained reporter thought that the maltreatment endangered the children or if a CPS investigation substantiated or indicated their maltreatment.

[32] In addition to the main study, the NIS–4 included several supplementary studies designed to enhance interpretations of NIS findings, such as surveys of CPS agencies. HHS is currently comparing the methodologies, including definitions, used by NIS-4 and NCANDS. This comparison analysis—which will not address child maltreatment fatalities—will be issued as a supplementary study to the NIS-4.

[33] Definitions of child abuse and neglect and procedures for responding to allegations of maltreatment are established by state legislative and departmental authority, according to HHS.

[34] In January 2008, CDC published definitions of child maltreatment and included recommended data elements designed to promote public health departments' voluntary use of consistent terminology for data collection related to child maltreatment. Reviewers and panelists involved in developing these definitions included NCANDS staff and consultants and the director of the National Center for Child Death Review. See CDC, National Center for Injury Prevention and Control (NCIPC), *Child Maltreatment Surveillance: Uniform Definitions for Public Health and Recommended Data Elements* (January 2008).

[35] The data-mapping process helps states define and align state data elements with NCANDS data elements and format. The process has been an integral part of state reporting since 1998, according to HHS officials.

[36] As HHS notes, NCANDS data are influenced by the states that report information over the years, and even small fluctuations in the data can affect the total numbers. The populations of the reporting states in fiscal year 2009 were different enough compared with the populations in fiscal year 2008 to affect both the national estimate and the national rate. See HHS, *Child Maltreatment 2009.*

[37] The term "circumstances" in this report refers to the factors surrounding and contributing to incidents of fatal child maltreatment. These factors include information on the child, the perpetrator, and the context for the child's death, such as its cause, location, date, type of maltreatment, and caregiver characteristics.

[38] For selected NCANDS data results on child fatalities, see app. II.

[39] In addition to data that states report to NCANDS, 32 states collected information on child maltreatment fatalities that were not reported to NCANDS in fiscal year 2009, according to our survey of state child welfare officials. See app. III for more information on data that states collected that were not reported to NCANDS.

[40] In commenting on a draft of this report, HHS noted that the annual *Child Maltreatment* report for 2013 will include additional analyses of caregiver risk factors of children who died and the total number of reported fatalities by state during the previous 5 years.

[41] The term "indicated" refers to a report disposition that concludes that maltreatment cannot be substantiated under state law or policy, but there is reason to suspect that the child may have been maltreated or was at risk of maltreatment. This is applicable only to states that distinguish between substantiated and indicated dispositions.

[42] In January 2005, the Office of the Assistant Secretary for Planning and Evaluation, HHS, issued a study on *Male Perpetrators of Child Maltreatment: Findings from NCANDS* utilizing an 18-state dataset of perpetrators identified by the CPS system during 2002. This study focused on perpetrators of child maltreatment generally but did not discuss child fatalities specifically. See U.S. Department of Health and Human Services, Office of the Assistant Secretary for Planning and Evaluation, *Male Perpetrators of Child Maltreatment: Findings from NCANDS* (Washington, D.C.: 2005).

[43] Unmarried partners pose higher risks of maltreatment: Compared with children living with married biological partners, those whose single parent had a live-in partner had more than eight times the rate of maltreatment overall, according to the NIS-4.

[44] Children with disabilities are likely undercounted since not every child receives a clinical diagnostic assessment from a CPS agency worker that is confirmed by a physician or other expert. NCANDS includes this as a limitation to its disability data.

[45] For selected results from our analysis of child maltreatment data in the CDR Reporting System, see app. II.

[46] Follow-up may include providing services to surviving family members, providing information to assist in prosecuting perpetrators, and developing recommendations to improve child protection systems. Many states received initial funding for child death review teams through CAPTA formula grants, commonly called Children's Justice Act grants, to improve the prosecution and handling of child abuse and neglect cases. (CAPTA § 107.)

[47] According to NCCDR, 49 states have a child death review program: 37 states have a state-level panel and teams in local communities, mostly at the county level; and 12 states have only state-level review teams.

[48] Although NCCDR is funded by HRSA, the Office of Management and Budget does not consider the NCCDR data reporting system a federal database because HRSA does not review or approve child death reviews and no data are submitted directly to HRSA.

[49] In defining maltreatment, NCCDR limits perpetrators to parents and caregivers, while NCANDS does not limit the definition in this way.

[50] In commenting on a draft of this report, HHS noted that NCCDR recently established a data dissemination plan to allow NCCDR data to be studied and published at the national level.

[51] For the purposes of this report, medical issues include those related to the determination of maltreatment by medical professionals, including identifying cases of abuse or neglect, and properly documenting those cases.

[52] According to CDC, shaken baby syndrome is a leading cause of child abuse deaths in the United States, and at least one of four babies who are violently shaken dies from this form of maltreatment. Although babies with shaken baby syndrome may display some outward signs, these injuries are not always visible.

[53] HHS *Child Maltreatment 2009* report.

[54] According to the International Association of Coroners and Medical Examiners, the cost of an autopsy ranges from several hundred dollars to several thousand, depending on the extent of the postmortem examination and other tests, such as X-rays, which incur additional costs.

[55] Committee on Identifying the Needs of the Forensic Sciences Community, National Research Council. S*trengthening Forensic Science in the United States: A Path Forward*. A special report prepared at the request of the Department of Justice. Washington, D. C.: August 2009.

[56] Forensic pathology is a subspecialty of medicine devoted to the investigation and physical examination of persons who die a sudden, unexpected, suspicious, or violent death.

[57] Training on death scene investigation—supported by the Department of Justice's (DOJ) Office of Juvenile Justice and Delinquency Prevention—is also available at the national level for professionals involved in the child death investigation process, such as medical personnel, law enforcement, and child welfare workers. This week-long, multidisciplinary training covers techniques for investigating child fatalities, including examples of common and uncommon fatal child maltreatment cases and injuries specific to children. Additionally, training and technical assistance resources for multidisciplinary professionals may be requested and funded through DOJ's Office for Victims of Crime's Training and Technical Assistance Center.

[58] Confidentiality and privacy issues include the 1996 Health Insurance Portability and Accountability Act's (HIPAA) privacy rule, which provides protections for personal health information. See generally 45 C.F.R. pt. 164, subpts. A and E (2010). In addition, states that receive CAPTA basic grants must provide assurance that they have a statewide program that includes provisions or methods to (1) maintain the confidentiality of all records and reports related to their child abuse and neglect investigations; (2) release information from these confidential records to any federal, state, or local government entity, or an agent of these entities that need this information to carry out their responsibilities under law to protect children from abuse and neglect; and (3) release to the public information

concerning a child abuse and neglect case when it resulted in the death (or near death) of a child.

[59] The NCANDS State Advisory Group is composed of members from Alaska, California, Connecticut, District of Columbia, Indiana, Kentucky, Louisiana, Massachusetts, Michigan, Missouri, New Mexico, New York, North Dakota, Oklahoma, Oregon, Puerto Rico, South Carolina, South Dakota, Tennessee, and Vermont.

[60] The goal of the National Resource Center for Child Welfare Data and Technology (NRC-CWDT) is to improve the quality of data reported to the federal government in the Adoption and Foster Care Analysis and Reporting System, NCANDS, Statewide Automated Child Welfare Systems, and the National Youth in Transition Database. In addition, according to HHS, the National Resource Center on Child Protective Services has often been called in after a child fatality has occurred to review state CPS systems and determine if the fatality could have been prevented. States may request on-site technical assistance through their Administration for Children and Families Regional Office.

[61] The HHS Office on Child Abuse and Neglect leads and coordinates the Federal Interagency Workgroup on Child Abuse and Neglect, which represents over 40 federal agencies. The overall goals of the workgroup are to provide a forum through which staff from relevant federal agencies can communicate and exchange ideas concerning child maltreatment-related programs and activities, to collect information about federal child maltreatment activities, and to provide a basis for collective action through which funding and resources can be maximized. However, HHS officials told us that the topic of child maltreatment fatalities has not often been discussed at these quarterly meetings.

[62] The Paperwork Reduction Act requires that federal agencies obtain OMB approval before collecting information from the public (such as forms, general questionnaires, surveys, instructions, and other types of collections). 44 U.S.C. § 3507.

[63] In Pennsylvania, we also met with county CPS officials from Franklin, Lycoming, Montgomery, and Sullivan counties.

[64] This analysis was conducted by NCCDR for our study using data for calendar year 2009. Results are based on data from 20 states.

[65] In addition to CPS records, documentation could include information on prior abuse obtained from law enforcement reports, medical records, or autopsy reports.

[66] The child could have died from maltreatment that occurred prior to placement in foster care, and not necessarily by maltreatment inflicted by the foster parent.

In: Child Fatalities Due to Maltreatment
Editors: V. Chapman and A. Burton
ISBN: 978-1-61942-342-8

Chapter 2

TESTIMONY OF THERESA M. COVINGTON NATIONAL CENTER FOR THE REVIEW AND PREVENTION OF CHILD DEATHS BEFORE THE COMMITTEE ON WAYS AND MEANS SUBCOMMITTEE ON HUMAN RESOURCES US HOUSE OF REPRESENTATIVES HEARING ON "CHILD DEATHS DUE TO MALTREATMENT" JULY 12, 2011[1]

Theresa M. Covington

Thank you Chairman Davis, Ranking Member Doggett and Members of the Subcommittee for providing me with this opportunity to speak to you about the tragedy of fatal child abuse.

I serve as the Director of the National Center for the Review and Prevention of Child Deaths, formerly known as the National Center for Child Death Review. We are based at the Michigan Public Health Institute. We are a resource center beginning our tenth year, funded through a cooperative

[1] This is an edited, reformatted and augmented version of a testimony before the Committee on Human Resources, dated July 2011.

agreement with the Maternal and Child Health Bureau within the Health Resources and Services Administration at HHS. Our center provides training and technical assistance to states as they work to conduct comprehensive and multidisciplinary case reviews of child deaths. Child Death Review (CDR) expanded to most states in the late 1990s, through training support from the Administration on Children and Families and OJJDP at the Department of Justice. In 2003, HRSA established funds for our national resource center, to encourage the focus on the prevention of deaths through the reviews. Today every state and Washington DC, with the exception of Idaho, has a CDR program in place but states vary greatly in their CDR structures, administrative homes, funding levels, and timing of reviews. Forty-four states have legislation requiring reviews and there is no national legislation requiring or supporting CDR. CAPTA legislation does however encourage death reviews of children known to the child welfare system through the citizen review process. Thirty-seven states support reviews at the county level with a state level advisory board that reviews these local findings to improve state policy and practice. Twelve states only have state-level review teams. Most states review deaths from a wide variety of causes including diseases, accidents, homicides and suicides-but all states review deaths from child abuse and neglect. All states review deaths from birth to age 18. There are two U. S. Healthy People 2020 Objectives especially related to CDR: *allstates and the District of Columbia will review 100% of allsudden and unexpected infant deaths and all deaths from external causes*-this would include child maltreatment.

Even those many states do not require participation on CDR, thousands of professionals regularly participate at CDR meetings to share case records from law enforcement, death investigators, social services, health care, public health, the courts, education, mental health and others in order to better understand why a child died and then to use that understanding to develop programs, policies and services to prevent future deaths. Most states review deaths from a wide variety of causes including diseases, accidents, homicides and suicides-but all states review deaths from child abuse and neglect. All states review deaths from birth to age 18.

As described in the just released GAO report to you, in 2005 our Center also built and now maintains the National Child Death Review Case Reporting System. The data is stored at the Michigan Public Health Institute. Thirty-nine states are now voluntarily enrolled in this on-line system-submitting comprehensive case reports on all of the deaths they review. This reporting tool allows for the collection of much more comprehensive information on child deaths than is available from any other single source-because it is a compilation of the information provided by many agencies at a review meeting, including vital records, and reports from medical examiners, law enforcement and child protective services. We have information on the child, their caregivers, supervisors, perpetrators, quality of the investigation, and the actual circumstances based on the cause of death and team recommendations for improvements to prevent other deaths. The report tool has over 1,800 data elements that can be answered by a team. We have also added additional questions for the seven states funded by the CDC Division of Reproductive Health's pilot of a national case registry for sudden and unexpected infant deaths (SUID). SUID deaths include those from SIDS, suffocation and undetermined causes and these can be almost impossible to distinguish at autopsy from a homicide caused by asphyxiation. The funded states include Colorado, Georgia, New Hampshire, Michigan, Minnesota, New Jersey and New Mexico. The CDC is contracting with our Center to assist states in improving their child death investigations and reporting on these mostly sleep-related infant deaths so that we can better understand and prevent them. With the CDC we are actively encouraging the use of the CDC's standard infant death investigation protocol. This protocol was developed by national experts through the leadership of the Division of Reproductive Health at the CDC, and they provided five training academies across the United States to build a cadre of trainers in states. You might be interested to know that we built the software for this system at the Michigan Public Health Institute, using funds from our core center grant of $450,000. We have continued to maintain the website, manage several thousand users, the data base and data storage all within these core funds-which are also used for all of our other Center activities. Our small staff of 3 people supports the center and the reporting system. States and local teams use the data for their own purposes and most states prepare annual reports. Data submitted into the reporting system is the property of states and we do not provide case identified data to anyone. We are just beginning to analyze national level data but have yet to extensively analyze the maltreatment data.

As of today, states have recorded 94,473 child deaths into the National CDR Case Reporting System. Teams reported that child abuse, child neglect or poor supervision was a factor in 7,894 or 8.3 percent of these deaths.

The GAO Report is right – significantly more children die from abuse and neglect than is reported through NCANDS, vital records or law enforcement databases alone. A number of studies have published this fact; including findings published in the American Public Health Association's Journal about the US Centers for Disease Control's child maltreatment surveillance project in seven states between 2001-2003. I was the principal investigator in Michigan. We found that in an average year, vital records reported 16 child abuse deaths; law enforcement records 26 deaths, child protective services 40 deaths. A high percentage of these deaths were only reported in one source and not another. However, after child death review and a synthesizing of all reporting sources, the number increased to over 100 deaths a year. This finding is troubling, especially considering that the GAO report found that 24 states reported to NCANDS only data from CPS. Other efforts have found similar outcomes.

Our Center assisted Clark County, Nevada which includes Las Vegas, conduct intensive reviews of seventy-nine deaths thought to be associated with abuse or neglect. OF these deaths, only six were coded on death certificates as maltreatment from physical abuse. Only nine had been substantiated as maltreatment by CPS. Following the review, an additional twenty-six deaths were identified as requiring CPS substantiation. A large number of deaths were not even reported to CPS because law enforcement and coroners felt that the family had suffered enough with the death of their child; or that it was a "bad accident" or that the parents did not intend to kill their children; or because there were no surviving siblings. And when CPS did take a report, more often than not they did not investigate for the same reasons. In the few cases they did investigate they did not substantiate. And when they did open an investigation, oftentimes they did not substantiate. The one area in which investigations were more routinely conducted and actions taken were deaths from serious physical abuse. But most of the deaths were from accidental injuries, or from serious medical complications of asthma, diabetes or childbirth-with non-compliance of treatment or substance use by the care givers. Overwhelmingly the reviews found that poor coordination during a death investigation among agencies can lead to this under-reporting and failure to address the abuse and neglect. The good news is that Clark County and the State of Nevada used the information discovered through these reviews to implement widespread improvements in their death investigation, CPS and judicial systems to better protect children.

We also have evidence of this undercounting across the nation by comparing the data available in state child death review annual reports, our child death review case reporting system data and NCANDS data. The following table includes data from available CDR state annual reports compared with data from NCANDS for the last year that state annual CDR was available as well as data for that same year submitted to the National CDR Case Reporting System.

Deaths due to neglect are especially underreported. These include those in which a caregiver *egregiously* failed to protect a child from known hazards or to provide care. These include, for example, drownings of infants and toddlers in bathtubs, house fires wherein children were left alone overnight, children left in cars on hot days, or infants suffocated while sleeping together with their intoxicated parent on couches or beds. Another area is medical neglect. In many cases these deaths are counted as deaths from natural, medical causes but a through case review may reveal that the caregivers failed to provide

State	**Number of Deaths by Abuse/Neglect Drawn From:**			
	NCANDS	**CDR database**	**State annual CDR report**	**Comments re state annual reports to CDR**
Arizona	11	23	51	For 2008
California	30	N/A	133	For 2001
Florida	156	N/A	192	2009. Not participating in CDR database
Georgia	60	22	77	2009
Iowa	6	3	7	For 2007
Kansas	10	N/A	13	For 2008. Not participating in CDR database.
Kentucky	22	N/A	28	For 2008, not participating in CDR data
Minnesota	16	N/A	19	For 2001
Missouri	39	N/A	109	2009. 33 of 109 are attributed to homicide by abuse; the 76 others are attributed to child abuse/neglect.
Nevada	17	5	37	For 2008
New Jersey	29	11	30	2008
Oklahoma	26	N/A	50	2006
Oregon	18	N/A	20	1999
Pennsylvania	40	10	98	2009. Includes death as a result of poor or absent supervision as well as death as a result of neglect
Washington	36 over the same 3 years	N/A	165 over 3 years	1999-2001: abuse/neglect "cited as a factor"

Compiled by National Center for the Review and Prevention of Child Deaths, July 2011

adequate care to keep the children healthy or alive. Examples include children who have manageable asthma or diabetes but caregivers fail to provide medication or to seek treatment when the child is critically ill.

I agree with the GAO findings on some of the reasons for the underreporting: lack of consistent definitions of maltreatment state to state and even within states; what Mississippi calls child abuse, Connecticut might call a sad accident or vice versa. There are inconsistencies across jurisdictions on how the determination of abuse and negle4ct is made and by whom- the CPS worker, the coroner, law enforcement, or the prosecutor? There are varying standards for criminal or civil charges of abuse or neglect. Community standards also vary widely across the U.S. influencing professional judgments. I have listened to many a CDR team member express frustration that a death will not be counted as abuse because the family has suffered enough, or "there but by the grace of God go I." Across the country I have listened to review teams describe very uncoordinated and/or incomplete investigations in child deaths-sometimes because resources are so limited for investigations and sometimes because investigators haven't been well trained. I have also been to many a review meeting in which the team members all agree that the child was killed by a caregiver but the prosecutor says he'll never get a jury to convict and thus no further action is taken.

On a positive note, we also know that by reviewing and understanding these deaths, communities and states are able to act on initiatives to prevent future deaths. That is why it is so important that we investigate, count and review these deaths accurately. I could spend all day here describing fantastic efforts implemented across the U.S. as a result of child death review. Some specific to the states you represent include: Kentucky has implemented new fire escape education for families because of deaths in which children died and adults survived. A number of states including North Dakota, Minnesota, Michigan, New York, Georgia and Lousisiana have implemented major public awareness' campaigns on shaken baby prevention and/or safe infant sleep awareness in part because of their reviews. North Dakota improved their death reporting policies to CPS as a result of reviews. Tennessee developed new services for high risk families, including evidence-based home visitation. In Texas, their state CDR recommended that all CPS caseworkers be trained in infant death investigation-CPS there is now systematicall y training caseworkers across the 254 Texas counties based on these recommendations. Washington State recently trained 150 law enforcement officers on child death investigations. A number of states have changed mandatory reporting policies to CPS, for example requiring reports even if there are no surviving siblings. Michigan published the results of six years of review findings and subsequent recommendations and improvements in outcomes for children. They found a significant correlation between recommendations implemented into practice and declines in deaths associated with the problems addressed in those recommendations. In other words, when the state took action to address the systems problems associated with child maltreatment deaths, they had a drop in deaths that had those systems problems. One example is deaths of children from abuse with multiple prior but unsubstantiated CPS reports. Michigan implemented a policy requiring investigation after any three reports to CPS following a number of deaths in which children died and were found to have multiple unsubstantiated reports. Another example is children dying who had histories of presenting to the emergency department with injuries but the ED did not report these injuries to CPS. The state instituted widespread training for ED health professionals on mandatory reporting, and now the state sees few child deaths with prior non-reported ED histories.

I agree with the GAO recommendations to improve the comprehensiveness, quality and use of national data on maltreatment deaths. In particular our Center looks forward to being part of the solution-working with ACF, NCANDS and our child death review teams to identify mechanisms to share and use our data from child death review to improve our data, our understanding of these deaths and to prevent other deaths. We hope that there will be federal action to develop standard definitions for fatal maltreatment in civil and criminal jurisdictions; action to address privacy and confidentiality barriers that prevent the sharing of information when such information is needed to keep a child or surviving siblings safe; and increased efforts that focus on children with serious injuries from maltreatment that are not yet fatal.

As a member of the National Coalition to End Child Abuse Deaths I also urge you to call for a National Commission as one part of the solution to study the complexities and offer national solutions to the issues presented in the GAO report.

But our states also need additional resources. Despite the fact that our nation is undergoing a severe budget crisis, we should not be a nation that fixes its budget crisis at the expense of abused and neglected children. Other than the $600,000 in funds allocated for *our* resource center, there is no dedicated funding to states for child death review or for the child death review case reporting system. Most states piecemeal their CDR programs together using state funds, Title V MCH block grant funds or CAPTA and Children's justice Act funds-never having enough to do justice to the children who have died. A bill was introduced in the last Congress and has been written this year but not yet introduced that will provide dedicated funding to states for child death review and improvements to child death investigations, especially those for sudden and unexplained infant deaths. And in addition to CDR, states certainly need emergency help for child protection as their resources dwindle while child abuse and neglect increases.

Our current CDR Case reporting system is rapidly becoming outdated and the software is fragile; but federal funds were not available to upgrade the software. Fortunately for our Center and the Case Reporting System's users, we have a new public-private partnership with Vantage Systems Inc., a private company known for its IT and engineering work at NASA's Goddard Space Flight Center. Vantage is donating its own staff and infrastructure to build a better version of our National CDR Case Reporting System. Vantage is doing this pro bono because in the words of their Vice President, Mike Ahan, "maybe our work can save one child's life." We anticipate receiving a complete software package from Vantage later this summer. Our Center and the technical support services at the Michigan Public Health Institute will work to launch this new version in January of 2012. It will have great improvements in functionality for states, including capacities to better link data with other sources, e.g. vital records, CPS and investigation records.

Children have no power or say in what happens to them. It is our responsibility and duty to protect them and use our knowledge and lessons learned from a child's death to prevent another death. Having comprehensive and reliable data on child deaths and using that data to save children should be the foundation of our child protection efforts. The bottom line for me, and I know for the thousands of child death review teams members who spend their time together sharing horribly sad stories of children, is that we need to do a much better job working together at the local, state and national level to address the underlying causes of child abuse and neglect; work better to investigate, respond, count and report on the deaths, and most importantly create solutions to keep kids safe, healthy, happy and alive.

Chairman Davis, Mr. Doggett and those of you on the this committee, tonight I ask that you think about the seven and maybe even eight or nine or ten children who died today because someone who is supposed to tuck them in at night killed them instead. And then tomorrow please use your power on this committee to take action to keep our children alive.

Thank you.

In: Child Fatalities Due to Maltreatment ISBN: 978-1-61942-342-8
Editors: V. Chapman and A. Burton

Chapter 3

TESTIMONY OF MICHAEL PETIT, PRESIDENT EVERY CHILD MATTERS EDUCATION FUND BEFORE THE COMMITTEE ON WAYS AND MEANS SUBCOMMITTEE ON HUMAN RESOURCES US HOUSE OF REPRESENTATIVES HEARING ON "CHILD DEATHS DUE TO MALTREATMENT" JULY 12, 2011[1]

Michael Petit

Chairman Davis, Ranking Member Doggett, Members of the Subcommittee, thank you for the opportunity to testify on this urgent issue. It is one in which I have been involved for 40 years, including the time that I served as Maine's health and human services commissioner, and while at the Child Welfare League of America.

According to official federal statistics, 13,856 children died from child abuse and neglect during the 2001-2009 period. Additionally, several studies

[1] This is an edited, reformatted and augmented version of a testimony before the Committee on Ways and Means Subcommittee on Human Resources, dated July 2011.

have concluded there actually is significant undercounting of maltreatment deaths, and that the true number may be several thousands more than reported.

Much can be done to reduce these child abuse and neglect deaths. There exists a vast body of knowledge about healthy child growth and development, including how to prevent abuse in the first place, and how to protect children from further harm if abuse should occur. But the sheer amount of child abuse and neglect in America—already more than 20 million reports of maltreatment made to government agencies in this decade—is certain evidence that, despite the best efforts of the many who work daily to address this problem, we continue to fall far short in applying our knowledge.

While the day to day direct responsibility for the protection of at-risk children rests with thousands of local and state child protection agencies, law enforcement, and courts across the country, their efforts could be greatly strengthened by expanding federal planning, coordination, and funding aimed at reducing child deaths.

Child Abuse Deaths Are Preventable. The President and Congress Must Elevate the Protection of Children to a National Priority if Children Facing Mortal Danger Are to be Protected

The official number of children killed from abuse or neglect nationwide in 2009 is 1,770. In 2001, the total was 1,300. Three-quarters of the children are under four.The current systems of child protection are stretched too thin to protect these children.

Between 2001-2009, the official number of child abuse and neglect fatalities was 13,856. The U.S. Department of Health and Human Services has reported an increasing number and rate of fatalities. In thousands of these cases, people reported the danger facing the child to authorities. For a variety of reasons— especially child protective agency budgets and staff capacity stretched dangerously thin in comparison to the problem—the response to these warnings failed the child. Now a harsh economy combined with a steadily weakened safety net in many states—including unprecedented slashes in child protection spending in some states— threaten to put even more children at risk.

The direct administration of protective services to children at risk of imminent harm properly rests with state and local governments. But with a long history of inadequate funding for child protection and severe budget crises at the state and local levels threatening public safety, the federal government alone possesses the authority and resources to ensure equal protection to children all across the country.

It remains a little known fact that the federal government already provides nearly half of the funds in the formal child welfare system and much of the statutory framework. The federal government is also legally obligated to evaluate each state's child protection performance and to prescribe recommendations for improvement. But, as presently constructed, neither federal funding nor federal oversights are at levels sufficient to protect all children who require it.

The Actual Number of Child Fatalities Is Unknown but Is Believed to be Much Higher than Official Statistics

Well-documented research suggests the number of children who die from abuse and neglect is considerably higher than official government statistics. Here's how the federal government defines maltreatment deaths:

> "Fatal child abuse may involve repeated abuse over a period of time (e.g., battered child syndrome), or it may Involve a single, impulsive incident (e.g., drowning, suffocating, or shaking a baby). In cases of fatal neglect, the child's death results not from anything the caregiver does, but from a caregiver's failure to act. The neglect may be chronic (e.g., extended malnourishment) or acute (e.g., an infant who drowns after being left unsupervised in the bathtub)."

Using this definition, several peer-reviewed studies conclude that there is a significant undercount of child maltreatment deaths. This is mainly due to what some researchers believe to be the improper classification of many maltreatment deaths as "unintentional injury death," deaths such as those caused by drowning, fire, suffocation, and poisoning. Upon examination of the circumstances underlying such deaths by forensic, medical and maltreatment experts—particularly if conducted by multi-disciplinary teams—the percentage of cases re-classified as maltreatment-related may comprise 50% or more of the unintentional injury deaths attributed to other causes on death certificates. The vast majority of these re-classified deaths are associated with inadequate supervision of children, often rising to the level of neglect.

If the research is correct about this "under-ascertainment" of maltreatment-related deaths, if it holds roughly true nationwide, then thousands of additional children should be included in the official maltreatment death toll from 2001-2009. What explains the undercount? There are a variety of reasons, including different state definitions of what constitutes a child abuse and neglect death, data collection methodologies, inconsistent record-keeping across the country, and who it is that actually determines the cause of death.

For example, a local child protective services agency opens a case involving child neglect. But because the mother agrees to treatment, the agency decides to leave the child home. However, the mother continues her drug use and one afternoon passes out in her apartment. Meanwhile, her two-year-old child plays unsupervised on a street and is struck by a car. In most states the death is recorded as a pedestrian accident, not the child neglect-related death that the federal definition would suggest it is.

A promising development in determining the amount of maltreatment deaths has been the creation of state child death review teams. In virtually all states there is a team which exists to review child deaths and determine their cause, including deaths from child abuse and neglect. The information resulting from this multidisciplinary team process provides invaluable data which can shape public health, law enforcement, and child welfare policy and practice. The teams vary in their capacity to conduct their activities. Some are well-funded and give each case the attention required; many don't have the necessary resources. The review teams agree on the need for stronger efforts to prevent child abuse and neglect deaths. In the words of one state's team manager: ÒFor conditions that are 100% preventable, we do a very poor and extremely fragmented job at preventing child maltreatment, as well as protecting those being maltreated."

Child Abuse and Neglect Fatalities Flow from Extensive Child Maltreatment in the U.S.

Nearly 20 million annual reports of abuse and neglect have been made to official state child protection agencies in this decade. And while 'only' a third or so of these reports were initially substantiated as abuse or neglect, it is often just a matter of time before many of the unsubstantiated cases also reveal themselves to be true as new report s involving the same family continue to be made to the child protection agency. There is no evidence which suggests that intentionally false reports alleging maltreatment are a serious issue. The reality is that child abuse and neglect in our culture are common.

Furthermore, state reporting to the federal government—required by law—remains uneven: since 2001, 24 states did not report child abuse and neglect numbers for at least one of the years in the Department of Health and Human Services annual Child Maltreatment report, and some did not report at all. Even without complete state data, the official numbers of children reported abused or neglected are staggering. Additionally, incidence studies of abuse and neglect conducted for the federal government suggest that the actual occurrences of maltreatment may be three times greater than the number of reports made to state child protection agencies.

Of the 721,646 children confirmed abused and neglected in 2007:

- 60% did not receive proper food, clothing, shelter, hygiene, education, medical care or protection.
- 13% suffered from multiple maltreatments.
- 11% were physically abused.
- 8% were sexually abused.
- 4% suffered from emotional abuse.
- 1% suffered from medical neglect.
- 4% suffered from other mistreatment such as abandonment, threats, and congenital drug addiction.
- 50% or more of child abuse and neglect cases are associated with alcohol or drug abuse by parents.

Of the millions of children reported abused or neglected each year, several thousand are in life threatening situations. The present systems of child protection successfully intervene in many of these situations, and further harm to a child is prevented. But for nearly 2,000 children, whatever response may be generated is too little, too late, and children die.

Many More American Children Die from Abuse and Neglect than do Children in other Advanced Countries

Among the richer democracies, the U.S. child abuse death rate is 3 times higher than Canada's, and 11 times higher than Italy's.

What accounts for the differences? Among other things, teen pregnancy, violent crime, imprisonment, and poverty rates are much lower in these countries. Further, their social policies in support of families are much greater and typically include child care, universal health insurance, paid parental leave, visiting nurses, and more—all things which together can prevent child abuse and neglect in the first place.

The U.S. invests only modestly in similar preventive measures compared to the needs of the most vulnerable families. This serious social policy lapse creates an environment where child abuse and neglect are common—where preventable maltreatment fatalities are inevitable.

It Is Largely an Accident of Geography Whether Abused or Neglected Children Receive the Full Protection They Need

As hard as they may try, no states are in full compliance with federal child welfare standards. No matter, state child protection reform efforts, often stemming from federal reviews and evaluations, have fueled many positive changes in state child protection practices in recent years.

But the combination of millions of children in harm's way and inadequate resources leaves many states stretched too thin to protect all children who need it. Accordingly, it is unlikely that states will come into compliance with all federal standards anytime soon, especially in view of severe state budget woes. But some states do protect children better than others. For example, in 2007 the child abuse and neglect fatality rate in the bottom state was 16 times that in the top state.

Although a clear correlation has not been established on how much states spend on child protective services and their child abuse and neglect death rates, states which do allocate more funds are more likely to investigate all abuse and neglect reports, not just some, because social workers have more manageable workloads. They also are more likely to retain staff; invest heavily in training; provide timely mental health, substance abuse treatment, and other services; and to prosecute serious abusers. Some states have much less capacity to conduct such activities, and state budget problems are weakening already under-funded systems of child protection. Such huge variations in capability among the states and their thousands of child protection offices across the country can translate directly into whether children live or die.

Many Child Protection Workers Frequently Lack the Resources and Training They Need

Child protection work is labor intensive, difficult, and emotionally stressful. The consequences of the decisions that child protection workers must make can be enormous: leave a child in harm's way, for example, or exercise powerful state authority that can result in the termination of parental rights. When trained and experienced staffs have access to experienced supervisors and to timely services such as mental health, substance abuse treatment, police back-up, and emergency shelter, children are much more likely to be protected, and abusive parents are much more likely to learn how to care for their children safely.

Recruiting and retaining highly trained social workers is a must. A major factor in retention is workload size. Children inevitably fall through the cracks when child protection workers have unmanageable workloads, leaving workers frustrated. Caseload ratios in some jurisdictions are as high as 60 or more, even while national standards recommend 12 or fewer cases per worker. Another factor in recruitment is compensation. Starting salaries under $30,000 for child protection workers are not uncommon, and rarely do they rise above $50,000—modest sums in view of the important jobs they are asked to do.

Further, while child protection workers are the most prominent "first responders" to child abuse and neglect, there are many others on the front lines who also may be involved, including education, law enforcement, and health professionals. Often, these groups lack training and support for fulfilling their own obligations to report abuse and neglect and to protect children.

To protect children at high risk of life-threatening abuse and neglect, the official child protective services agencies and law enforcement must collaborate. Child protective workers are best able to focus on the needs of the child, and law enforcement personnel are essential when confronting serious abusers. Written protocols and joint training between child protective services and law enforcement are essential for protecting children. Such collaborative efforts are much better developed in some jurisdictions than others, including those served by children's advocacy centers.

Restrictive Confidentiality Laws Shield the Press, Elected Officials and the Public from Shortcomings in the Child Protection System

Originally intended to protect living child victims from publicity, confidentiality laws have become a hindrance to a better public understanding of child abuse and neglect fatalities. Sometimes used to shield the public from the details of a child's death, confidentiality laws also interfere with journalists gathering and reporting facts about the incident. Even lawmakers are sometimes denied access to information surrounding an individual case, information that is critical to strengthening the child protection system. The withholding of such information benefits no one.

Stories about child abuse and neglect deaths are often reported in local papers, especially if a child's situation was brought to the attention of authorities. Frequently, however, these reports reveal little about how the formal child protection system performed in a fatality case. Instead they may focus on the seeming inadequacy of the child protective worker in the case, and often they prompt a call for both the worker and agency administrator to be fired. This response does little to address the underlying systemic problem.

The national press generally limits its maltreatment coverage to the most sensational child deaths. It provides virtually no press coverage of the federal government's role in the prevention of child abuse and neglect fatalities. And it is rare to see members of Congress or senior Administration officials speaking to the issue.

Stopping Child Abuse and Neglect Fatalities Requires Fighting Child Poverty

While strengthening the formal child protective services system has the highest immediate promise for safeguarding children in dangerous situations, there are millions of children in marginal homes who are at daily risk of harm. Reducing this risk will reduce fatalities—and the need for protection in the first place. Reducing risk also poses an enormous economic challenge because, while child abuse occurs in all socioeconomic ranks, it lands hardest on children in the poorest families. In fact, poverty is the single best predictor of child abuse and neglect, and no wonder in view of the family stress often accompanying poverty. One study found that a child living in a family with an annual income of $15,000 or less was 22 times more likely to be abused than one in a family with an income of $30,000 or more.

One in five American children, over 14 million, still lives in poverty. Conditions that are still widespread in the U.S., i.e., teen parenthood, violence, mental illness, substance abuse, imprisonment, unemployment, low education, and poor housing, are all disproportionately associated with poverty and often wreak havoc on poor families and children.

Most fatality victims are very young and very poor. In 2007, 75% were four or younger, and almost half were under age one. As noted in the federal Department of Health and Human Services' report Child Abuse and Neglect Fatalities: Statistics and Interventions, "these children are the most vulnerable for many reasons, including their dependency, small size, and inability to defend themselves." Further, 70% of the fatalities involved a parent as perpetrator. And often the abuser is a poor "...young adultÉ without a high school diplomaÉ depressedÉ [who] has experienced violence first hand."

We know a great deal about preventing abuse and neglect and stopping related fatalities. When provided with support services and appropriate supervision, the vast majority of potentially abusive and neglectful parents can learn to safely care for their children. And many abused children who get help are resilient enough to overcome their history. But for many, the outcome is predictable: when childhood goes wrong, adulthood goes wrong, and the sad story of abuse, including death, repeats itself from one generation of troubled families to the next.

Children at Grave Risk of being Killed Require Protection from Their Government

We need a national approach for protecting children because of the heavy toll exacted from the nation caused by child abuse and neglect—thousands killed, millions of lives ruined, costs of more than $100 billion a year.

While it is too late to help the children shown in this report, we can honor their memories by vowing to protect every child in danger.

Yet even with broad public support for protecting every child from harm, the nation's present commitment of resources, laws, and policies is too little.

We can overcome inadequate funding for child protective services and wide variations in capacity among states only by enacting federal policy committed to protecting children no matter where they live.

CALL TO ACTION: STOP CHILD ABUSE AND NEGLECT DEATHS

A National Commission to End Child Abuse and Neglect Fatalities should be created by Congress. Building upon the best of current child protection systems, it should recommend a national strategy for stopping maltreatment deaths.

- Current levels of federal spending are far below the level needed to protect all children at imminent risk of harm. $3 billion to $5 billion in additional funds are required, for example, to allow child protective workers and other frontline personnel to have smaller caseloads and better training, and to provide a wide array of public health and social services to help at risk families.
- In consideration of expanded federal spending, states should be required to adopt national standards, drawn from existing best practices and policy, for protecting children.
- Congress should modify confidentiality laws to allow policy makers, the press, and the public to understand better what protection policies and practices need to be improved in the aftermath of a child's death.
- The Department of Health and Human Services should standardize definitions and methodologies used to collect data related to maltreatment deaths and should require states to provide such data in order to receive federal funds. Further, state child death review teams should be adequately funded.
- The Department of Health and Human Services, in cooperation with state child protective and public health agencies, should conduct a public education campaign to encourage reporting of child abuse and neglect, and to enlist communities in the protection of children.
- To better protect children at imminent risk of severe harm, the federal government, led by the Departments of Justice and Health and Human Services, and in cooperation with states, should adopt a model protocol for assuring that civil and criminal legal proceedings are

closely coordinated between child protection and law enforcement agencies.

In: Child Fatalities Due to Maltreatment
Editors: V. Chapman and A. Burton
ISBN: 978-1-61942-342-8

Chapter 4

TESTIMONY OF CAROLE JENNY, MD, MBA, COMMITTEE ON WAYS AND MEANS SUBCOMMITTEE ON HUMAN RESOURCES, U.S. HOUSE OF REPRESENTATIVES, HEARING ON CHILD DEATHS DUE TO MALTREATMENT, JULY 12, 2011[1]

Carole Jenny

Chairman Davis, Ranking Member Doggett, and Members of the Subcommittee, I thank you for the opportunity to testify on child deaths due to maltreatment. I am a Professor of Pediatrics at Brown Medical School and the Director of the Child Protection Program at Hasbro Children's Hospital in Providence, Rhode Island. I have provided medical care for abused and neglected children for over 28 years. I have a unique perspective on this issue because I believe I am the only person in this room who has often stood at the bedside in the emergency department or in the intensive care unit and actually witnessed the deaths of infants and children from maltreatment.

When the death of a child is a result of abuse or neglect, a sad event becomes an immense tragedy.[1] This was certainly seen most recently in the

---

[1] This is an edited, reformatted and augmented version of a testimony before the Committee on Ways and Means Subcomittee on Human Resources, dated July 2011.

public outcry over the death of Kaylee Anthony, a previously healthy, happy toddler.

The 1,700 yearly child maltreatment deaths reported by the National Child Abuse and Neglect Data System are just the tip of the iceberg.[2] As the GAO report points out, counting and tracking the number of deaths from maltreatment is challenging. Sometimes it is very difficult to distinguish between accidental and non-accidental death. For example, when a child is purposely suffocated with a pillow or a plastic bag, it can be impossible to distinguish this from a death by natural causes. In addition, many deaths from neglect are not counted as such. In Rhode Island a 3-year-old was told by his drunken father to go across a busy street to retrieve a discarded lamp from a neighbor's trash. He was hit by a car and killed, and his death was ruled an accident. And what about deaths caused by the late effects of maltreatment? If a teenaged survivor of horrific sexual abuse commits suicide because of her severe depression and post-traumatic stress, is that considered a child abuse death? In my opinion the root cause of death in that case is child maltreatment.

My interest is in providing more accurate primary data to the agencies that track child maltreatment deaths. These agencies cannot perform well if the cases they review have not been adequately investigated. The pediatric profession has recently made a giant leap in improving this process. The American Board of Pediatrics has established the board certified pediatric subspecialty of Child Abuse Pediatrics.[3] These pediatricians complete an additional 3 years of fellowship training in child maltreatment, becoming experts in the recognition, diagnosis, treatment and prevention of child maltreatment. When a child does die from abuse or neglect, these pediatricians can help police, forensic, and social service agencies make the correct diagnosis by doing the appropriate medical work up in the hospital and by ruling out conditions that mimic abuse or neglect.

There is currently no Federal support for training pediatric subspecialists in Child Abuse Pediatrics. We need to expand the availability of fellowships to make sure that these doctors are available to *all* hospitals around the country that care for children. The National Association of Children's Hospitals and Related Institutions has published recommended guidelines for the establishment of Child Protection Teams at all children's hospitals,[4] but there are not enough trained, board certified pediatric specialists in the field to do provide this expertise.

Another way to increase the accurate counting of child maltreatment deaths is to increase the resources available to medical examiners and coroners and to support their performance of quality death investigations. Multiple studies have shown that only about half of child maltreatment deaths are actually recognized and recorded on death certificates and in state vital statistics.[5-7]

In summary, in addition to improving our methods of *counting* child maltreatment deaths, we need to improve our ability to *recognize* and *discern* when a death is due to child maltreatment. And, if we have the resources to diagnose abuse and neglect and provide the necessary treatment and services to children and families, we can actually *prevent* the ultimate worst outcome, the death of a child. It is important to note that strengthening the quality of medical and death investigations in child abuse cases adds another protective factor. That is, we will be better able to protect innocent parents from allegations of child abuse and neglect, and to preserve and promote families.

This testimony represents the opinion of Dr. Carole Jenny and are not attributed to any organization.

REFERENCES

[1] Jenny, C. & Isaac, R. (2006). The relation between child death and child ma ltreatment. *Archives of Disease in Childhood*, *91*, 265-269.

[2] United States Government Accountability Office. Report to the Chairman, Committee and Ways and Means, House of Representatives: Child Maltreatment: Strengthening National Data on Child Fatalities Could Aid in Prevention. GAO-11-599, July 2011.

[3] Block, R. W. & Palusci, V. J. (2006). Child Abuse Pediatrics: A new pediatric subspecialty. *Journal of Pediatrics*, *48*, 711-712.

[4] National Association of Children's Hospital and Related Institutions. *Defining the Children's Hospital Role in Child Maltreatment.* Washington, DC, July (2006). Available online at https://www.childrens hospitals.net/AM/Template.cfm?Section=Search3&content=2005child_a buse_survey&template=/cm/contentdisplay.cfm&contentfileid=8173. Accessed July 10, 2011.

[5] Crume, T. L., DiGuiseppi, C., Byers, T., Sirotnak, A. P. & Garrett, C. J. (2002) Underascertainment of child maltreatment fatalities by death certificates, 1990-1998, *Pediatrics*, *110*, e1 8.

[6] Herman-Giddens, M. E., Brown, G., Verbiest, S., Carlson, P. J., Hooton, E. G., Howell. E. & Butts, J. (1999). Underascertainment of child abuse

mortality in the United States. *Journal of the American Medical Association*, 282, 463-467.

[7] Ewigman, B., Kivlahan, C. & Land, G. (1993). The Missouri child fatality study: Underreporting of maltreatment fatalities among children younger than five years of age, 1983 through 1986. *Pediatrics*, *91*, 330-337.

In: Child Fatalities Due to Maltreatment
Editors: V. Chapman and A. Burton
ISBN: 978-1-61942-342-8

Chapter 5

TESTIMONY OF JANE MCCLURE BURSTAIN, PH.D., SENIOR POLICY ANALYST, CENTER FOR PUBLIC POLICY PRIORITIES, BEFORE THE SUBCOMMITTEE ON HUMAN RESOURCES, HEARING ON "CHILD DEATHS DUE TO MALTREATMENT"[1]

Jane Burstain

Chairman Davis, Ranking Member Doggett and members of the Subcommittee, thank you for this opportunity to testify about the important issue of child maltreatment deaths. I have worked in the child welfare arena for more than a decade. In 1998, I left my civil litigation practice and started working as an attorney for the Children's Law Center in Los Angeles (CLC-LA) representing thousands of children over my tenure there. After working at CLC-LA for almost six years, I became interested in taking my experience working with children and families and translating it into systemic improvement. I earned a PhD in policy analysis at the Pardee RAND Graduate School, writing my dissertation on improving outcomes for teenage mothers in the child welfare system. After receiving my PhD in 2008, I came to work at

[1] This is an edited, reformatted and augmented version of a testimony before the subcommittee on Human Resources, dated July 2011.

the Center for Public Policy Priorities, a non-profit, nonpartisan think tank based in Austin, Texas that is committed to improving public policy to better the economic and social condition of low- to moderate-income Texans. At the Center, I work on child welfare policy and budget issues. I conduct research, participate in state and national coalitions and educate policy makers on how to create better outcomes for children and families.

I think you would agree that even one child maltreatment death is too many. But in 2009,[1] every single day more than 4 children were reported to have died from abuse or neglect in the United States.[2] And since not every state reports on child maltreatment deaths and some states that do report may not be capturing all such deaths, the actual number is probably even higher. Having quality, comprehensive and consistent data from the states regarding child maltreatment deaths is an important step in understanding why such deaths are happening and what can be done to prevent them.

While improving data collection and reporting procedures is important, it can take time and resources to accomplish. But we don't have to wait for the data to be perfect before we can act. The data we have now, even though limited, shows that states with a higher rate of child maltreatment deaths also have higher rates of child poverty and teen births. As families struggle and stress levels rise, child maltreatment becomes more of a risk. If we want to address this problem, we need to invest in our families and the future of our children. To cut programs that support struggling families in tough economic times is the very definition of penny-wise and pound foolish and is a choice our children will pay for with their lives.

Some States Have Significantly Higher Reported Child Maltreatment Death Rates

There is significant variation among the states with respect reporting deaths from child maltreatment. Some states do not report at all,[3] some states report that they have no child maltreatment deaths[4] and for the other states, total numbers range from 1 up to 279.[5]

Even taking the numbers at face value, with the differences in population size among the states, a comparison based on the total number of deaths is not always useful. Texas may have more reported child maltreatment deaths than Nevada, but it also has a significantly larger child population.

To look at the number of deaths in context, a rate that takes into account differences in population size must be used. For child maltreatment deaths, the rate used is the number of deaths per 100,000 children in the population. For example, Texas reported 279 child maltreatment deaths in 2009, which translates into a rate of about 4 deaths for every 100,000 children in its population. In contrast, Nevada reported only 29 child maltreatment deaths in 2009, but with its smaller child population, it actually has a slightly higher rate than Texas of 4.26 deaths for every 100,000 children.

Even looking at reported child maltreatment death rates, however, there still is significant variation among the states. And over the years, the child maltreatment death rate ranking among the states has changed, although some states like Texas consistently have higher rates than the average.

SOME STATES WITH HIGHER RATES SEEM TO HAVE A MORE ROBUST DATA COLLECTION AND REPORTING SYSTEM

Although the federal government collects child maltreatment data from the states, not all states report child maltreatment fatalities.[6] And even among the states that do report, there is significant variation in how they define, investigate and report when a child's death results from maltreatment, with some systems seeming more robust than others.

Some states have a broader definition of abuse and neglect and so may be more likely to identify a child's death as resulting from maltreatment. For example, 18 states include a parent's drug use in its definition of child maltreatment,[7] while the others do not.

The procedures for investigating whether a child's death is from maltreatment vary among the states as well. Although virtually every state has some sort of process for reviewing child deaths,[8] 30 of them have local involvement in their child death review process while the process in the other states is conducted solely at the state level.[9] Input from the communities in which the deaths occur may allow those states with local involvement to better investigate and identify when a death is from abuse or neglect.

Some states also have special investigative procedures that must be followed in a child death that may increase the accuracy of a child death evaluation. For example, in Texas, all deaths of children under the age of 6 must be reported to the county medical examiner who must conduct an inquest to determine whether the death is from abuse or neglect.[10] 30 other states also have some sort of special reporting procedures for suspicious child deaths.[11]

Finally, the 39 states that have a centralized child welfare system and database may have a more comprehensive and accurate data collection and reporting system for child maltreatment deaths compared to states with a decentralized, county-run system.[12] For example, Texas has a centralized system and reports data on child maltreatment deaths both at an individual case and an aggregate level. In contrast, California, with its decentralized, county-run system, only reports data on an aggregate level with no case-level details.

Looking at the characteristics together, only five states have all four characteristics (parental substance abuse in maltreatment definition, local involvement in death review, special investigative requirements and a state-run child welfare system): Florida, Illinois, Indiana, South Dakota, and Texas. And, collectively, these states have a higher rate of child abuse and neglect deaths as compared to other states.[13] This suggests that the higher rate of child maltreatment deaths in some states may not be because more deaths are occurring but, rather, because the state is doing a better job in investigating and reporting such deaths. In other words, it is likely that some states are underreporting and so the problem is probably even bigger than we think.

Improving the quality and consistency of available data about child maltreatment deaths, however, can be difficult. Increasing the quality of data collection and investigative procedures would require states to dedicate additional funding and resources which they simply may not have. Ensuring consistency is also problematic. Even if there were a national definition of maltreatment and some guidelines on how to classify child deaths, there may not always be consistent determinations. Determining whether maltreatment caused a child's death will always involve some level of subjective judgment and be affected by the resources dedicated to the investigation, especially when the death was accidental rather than intentional. For example, when a child dies from an accidental drowning, one state may carefully review the circumstances and conclude that the parent failed to appropriately supervise the child, classifying the death as from neglect. Another state investigating the same circumstances, however, may simply classify it as accidental and not even investigate the possibility of neglect.

STATES WITH HIGHER RATES OF CHILD MALTREATMENT DEATHS ALSO HAVE HIGHER RATES OF RISK FACTORS FOR CHILD ABUSE AND NEGLECT

As discussed above, a more robust data collection and reporting system may explain why some states have a higher child maltreatment death rate. But it does not fully explain the variation because even among the states with a robust system, there are differences. In 2009, Texas' child maltreatment death rate was 4.05 per 100,000 children while the average rate for the other robust system states (Florida, Illinois, Indiana and South Dakota) was statistically significantly lower at 3.1 per 100,000 children.

As discussed below, part of the differences in child maltreatment death rates appear to be related to risk factors that are more prevalent in certain states.

States with a High Child Poverty Rate Have a Higher Rate of Child Maltreatment Deaths[14]

Poverty is a consistent predictor of abuse and neglect. Children in families with an annual income of less than $15,000 are 14 times more likely to be abused and 44 times more likely to be neglected as compared to children in families with an annual income of $30,000 or more.[15] And, on average, states with high child poverty (defined as at or above 20 percent of the overall child population)[16] had a child maltreatment death rate that was 43 percent higher than states with lower child poverty.[17]

States with a High Teen Birth Rate Have a Higher Rate of Child Maltreatment Deaths[18]

Children with young mothers are at a higher risk of maltreatment.[19] And, on average, states with a high teen birth rate (defined as at or above 53 births per 1,000 teenaged females[20]) had a child maltreatment death rate that was 61 percent higher than states with a lower teen birth rate.[21]

Support for Programs that Help Alleviate Child Abuse and Neglect Risk Factors Are Needed Now, More than Ever

With the Great Recession and continued high unemployment, more families have been pushed into poverty. As compared to 2008, the number and percentage of children living in poverty increased nationally and in virtually every state in 2009, in some cases by up to 40 percent.[22]

And although the national teen birth rate has dropped in recent years, some states still struggle with the problem. In Texas, the teen birth rate has remained high for the last several years at around 63 births per 1,000 teenaged females so that in 2008, there were more than 55,000 births to girls younger than 20.[23]

In sum, the number of children at risk for child maltreatment continues to grow. To ensure that this trend does not translate into more child maltreatment deaths, Congress needs to ensure continued support and funding for programs that address risk factors.

Congress Needs to Ensure Continued Funding for Direct Child Abuse and Neglect Services

Despite an increase in the number of families at-risk for abuse and neglect, the number of children receiving prevention services has declined in 16 states.[24] As states grapple with huge revenue shortfalls, prevention programs are often the first casualties of the budget axe. In Texas, the legislature just passed a budget that cut child abuse and neglect prevention funding by 44 percent.[25] That means that in a state with more than 1.6 million children in poverty and at risk for maltreatment, only 6,000 will receive prevention services annually.[26]

Budgets are so tight that states are even cutting services to children who have been subjected to abuse and neglect. In 2008, an average of 63 percent of child maltreatment victims nationwide received services to address the family's problems. In 2009, the rate dropped to less than 60 percent and, in some states, the rate was so low that fewer than 1 in 3 child abuse and neglect victims received any such services.[27]

To avoid any further cuts, Congress must ensure that federal funding that supports child abuse and neglect services continues and is not cut. For example, funding under Title IV-B of the Social Security Act is the primary support in many states for child abuse and neglect prevention services. In 2009, Promoting Safe and Stable Families (PSSF) funding paid for more than 30 percent of prevention services nationwide and in 8 states[28], PSSF accounted for more than 50 percent of such services.[29] Funding for home visitation programs provided under the Patient Protection and Affordable Care Act is important as well. Studies have shown that such programs improve parenting and child health and safety and, in some cases, reduce maltreatment, even among the high risk population of adolescent mothers.[30]

Congress should also create a new Title IV-E waiver program so states can pilot more flexible ways to use dedicated child welfare federal funds to keep children at risk of child maltreatment safe at home instead of languishing in the more expensive and less optimal alternative of foster care. A detailed discussion of why Title IV-E waivers are necessary is contained in my recent written testimony to the U.S. Senate Committee on Finance at the hearing on Innovations in Child Welfare Waivers: Starting the Pathway to Reform.[31]

Support for Subsidized Early Education and other Child Care for Low Income, Working Families Needs to Continue

Several studies have demonstrated that Head Start and other subsidized early education and child care programs have been successful in reducing aggressive parenting behavior that can escalate into child abuse.[32] And one study in Chicago showed that young children from disadvantaged neighborhoods who participated in a child care program had 50 percent fewer court petitions related to maltreatment compared to children in similar neighborhoods that did not have the program.[33]

Some states also use child care to keep children who have already been subjected to abuse and neglect safe in their own homes. In Texas in state fiscal 2010, the state child welfare agency used subsidized day care to keep an estimated 17,000 young child maltreatment victims safe in their own home in lieu of removal.[34] Such options are not only better for the child but cheaper for the state. In Texas, foster care costs about $1,900/month while subsidized day care is less than $600/month.

Getting children out of the home and into day care helps relieve parental stress, gives parents non-physical models for discipline and makes the children more visible to potential reporters so problems can be identified before they escalate into something serious. But like prevention programs, funding for early education and child care has fallen victim to the budget axe. In Texas' most recent budget, the Legislature cut grants to support pre-kindergarten by 100 percent, cut funding for subsidized child care for at-risk children by 18 percent[35] and cut protective day care service levels by 16 percent.[36]

The recent cuts at the state level make funding from the federal Child Care Development Block Grant more important than ever as it is often the primary funding stream for such services. In Texas in 2010, 46 percent of day care for at-risk children and 50 percent of protective day care was funded through the Child Care Development Block Grant.[37]

The Supplemental Temporary Assistance to Needy Families Grant Needs to be Reauthorized

The supplemental Temporary Assistance to Needy Families grant was created specifically to help states with high poverty rates, which are the very same states that also have high child maltreatment death rates. Given the cuts that states have already implemented, reauthorizing this funding will help ensure that these programs are better protected in the future.

Expanded Health Insurance Options for Adults Will Help Alleviate Abuse and Neglect Risk Factors by Providing Access to Mental Health and Substance Abuse Treatment

Substance abuse is a significant risk factor for child abuse and neglect. When parents abuse substances, they pay less attention to their children which may result in more accidents or a lack of necessary medical care.[38] They are more likely to use harsh parenting styles and leave their children unattended and have other problems such as domestic violence, single-parenthood and depression, all of which may increase the likelihood of maltreatment.[39] Mental illness, which often co-occurs with substance abuse, also interferes with parenting and is a risk factor for child maltreatment.[40]

But most adults living in poverty have no way of obtaining health insurance and so lack access to substance abuse and mental health treatment. In Texas alone, 5 million adults age 19 to 64 are uninsured, the majority of whom are under 400 percent of the federal poverty limit.[41] Starting in 2014, however, under the Patient Protection and Affordable Care Act, these adults will be eligible for health insurance either through Medicaid or the Health Insurance Exchange and so will be able to access services and treatment.[42]

Access to appropriate mental health treatment such as counseling is especially important as at least one study found that parents who have insight into their mental health problems had less problematic parenting behavior and a lower risk of child maltreatment.[43]

CONCLUSION

With the Great Recession, more families have been pushed into poverty. As families struggle and stress levels rise, more kids are at risk of child maltreatment. If we want to address this problem, we need to invest in our families and the future of our children. If we don't, our children will pay for it with their lives. To cut programs that support struggling families just when they need it the most is the very definition of penny-wise and pound foolish.

At the same time, we need to work on getting quality, comprehensive and consistent data from the states regarding child maltreatment deaths so we can better understand why such deaths are happening and what else can be done to prevent them.

Respectfully submitted,

Jane Burstain, PhD
Senior Policy Analyst
Center for Public Policy Priorities

The Center for Public Policy Priorities is a nonpartisan policy institute committed to improving public policy to better the economic and social condition of low- to moderate-income Texans. We pursue this mission to achieve our vision for a BETTER TEXAS™.

End Notes

[1] Unless otherwise noted, all years refer to the federal fiscal year.

[2] Unless otherwise noted, all data regarding child maltreatment deaths is from the *Child Maltreatment* report published annually by the U.S. Department of Health and Human Services, Administration for Children and Families, Administration on Children, Youth and Families, Children's Bureau.

[3] In 2009, Alaska, Massachusetts, and North Carolina.

[4] For 2009, Montana and Wyoming.

[5] For2009.

[6] For federal fiscal year 2009, Alaska, Massachusetts and North Carolina did not report child abuse and neglect fatalities to the federal government.

[7] Arkansas, Colorado, Florida, Illinois, Indiana, Minnesota, North Dakota, South Carolina, South Dakota, Virginia and the District of Columbia include pre-natal drug exposure in their definition of abuse and neglect. California, Iowa, Kentucky, Minnesota, New York, Rhode Island and Texas include a parent's drug use in the definition of abuse and neglect to the extent it impairs the ability to care for the child. *Parental Drug Use as Child Abuse.* Child Welfare Information Gateway. May 2009. Available at: http://www.childwelfare.gov/ systemwide/laws_policies/statutes/drugexposed.cfm. Accessed on December 1, 2009.

[8] Idaho does not currently have a working program. National MCH Center for Child Death Review, State Spotlight-Idaho. Last updated February 2008. Available at: http://www.childdeathreview.org/spotlightID.htm. Accessed on July 8, 2011.

[9] Using state program descriptions from the National MCH Center for Child Death Review, State Spotlights (Available at: http://www.childdeathreview.org/state.htm. Accessed on November 10, 2009), local involvement is defined as reviews conducted solely at a local level, reviews conducted at both the state and local level and reviews conducted at a local level with state oversight. States with local involvement include: Alabama, Arizona, California, Colorado, Delaware, Florida, Georgia, Hawaii, Illinois, Indiana, Kentucky, Louisiana, Maryland, Massachusetts, Michigan, Missouri, Montana, Nevada, New Jersey, New York, Ohio, Oklahoma, Oregon, Pennsylvania, South Dakota, Texas, Vermont, Virginia, Washington, Wisconsin and Wyoming.

[10] Texas Family Code §§264.513-14.

[11] In addition to Texas, Arkansas, California, Colorado, Connecticut, Florida, Illinois, Indiana, Kansas, Louisiana, Maine, Massachusetts, Michigan, Minnesota, Missouri, Montana, Nevada, New York, North Carolina, Ohio, Pennsylvania, Rhode Island, South Carolina, South Dakota, Tennessee, Utah, Virginia, Washington, West Virginia, Wisconsin, Wyoming and Puerto Rico all have special reporting procedures for suspicious child deaths. *Making and Screening Reports of Child Abuse and Neglect*. Child Welfare Information Gateway. Current through January 2009. Available at: *http://www.childwelfare.gov/ systemwide/laws* policies/statutes/repproc.pdf. Accessed on July 8, 2011.

[12] 13 states have a county-administered system: California, Colorado, Georgia, Maryland, Minnesota, Nevada, New York, North Carolina, North Dakota, Ohio, Pennsylvania, Virginia and Wisconsin. *National Study of Child Protective Services Systems and Reform Efforts: Review of State CPS Policy.* U.S. Department of Health and Human Services Office of the Assistant Secretary for Planning and Evaluation and Administration for Children and Families Administration on Children, Youth and Families Children's Bureau. April 2003. Available at: *http://aspe.hhs.gov/hsp/cpsstatus03/state.* (Accessed on July 8, 2011).

[13] Burstain JM. *Child Abuse and Neglect Deaths in Texas.* Center for Public Policy Priorities. December 2009.

[14] Based on an ordinary least squares regression of child poverty on the child death rate and using a p-value of .05 to determine significance. Using data from 2007, child poverty was defined as an indicator with 1 meaning that a sta te had a rate at or above the 75percentile. Data on child poverty derived from the Annie E. Casey KIDS Count Data Center. Available at: http://datacenter.kidscount.org/data/acrossstates/Rankings.aspx?ind=45 (Accessed on October 30, 2009).

[15] Sedlack AJ, Broadhurst DD. *Executive Summary of Third National Incidence Study of Child Abuse and Neglect.* Administration of Children and Families. 1996. Available at: http://www.childwelfare.gov/pubs/statsinfo/nis3.cfm#top.. (Accessed on October 30, 2009).

[16] States with child poverty rates at or above 20 percent in 2007 include: Alabama, Arizona, Arkansas, Georgia, Kentucky, Louisiana, Mississippi, New Mexico, North Carolina, Oklahoma, Tennessee, Texas and West Virginia.

[17] Death rate was 2.51 for high poverty states versus 1.77 for other states. β =.74. The same effect was found using an indicator for states at or above the 75th percentile for: (1) children in extreme poverty (defined as an annual income of 50% or less than the federal poverty line) β =.80; and (2) children under 5 living in poverty β =.80.

[18] Based on an ordinary least squares regression of the teen birth rate on the child death rate and using a p-value of .05 to determine significance. Using data from 2006, teen birth rate was defined as an indicator with 1 meaning that a state had a rate at or above the 75percentile. Data on teen birth rates derived from the Annie E. Casey KIDS Count Data Center. Available at: http://datacenter.kidscount.org/data/acrossstates/Rankings.aspx?ind=45 (Accessed on October 30, 2009).

[19] Stiffman NM, et al. *Household Composition and Risk ofFatal Child Maltreatment.* Pediatrics 109(4):61 5-621. April 2002.

[20] Based on teens ages 15-19. Data derived from Annie E. Casey Kids Count Data Center. Available at: http://datacenter.kidscount.org/data/acrossstates/Rankings.aspx?ind=2. (Accessed on October 30, 2009). States with a high teen birth rate include: Alabama, Arizona, Arkansas, Georgia, Kentucky, Louisiana, Mississippi, Nevada, New Mexico, Oklahoma, Tennessee and Texas.

[21] β =.87.

[22] Annie E. Casey KIDS Count Data Center. Available at: *http://datacenter.kidscount.org/data/acrossstates/Rankings.aspx?ind=45* (Accessed on July 5,2011). The percentage of children living in poverty increased in Hawaii from 10 percent in 2008 to 14 percent in 2009.

[23] Teen birth data derived from Annie E. Casey Kids Count Data Center. Available at: http://datacenter.kidscount.org/data/acrossstates/Rankings.aspx?ind=2(Accessed on July 5, 2011).

[24] Comparing 2009 to 2008. States with declines are: Alaska, Arizona, Delaware, Georgia, Idaho, Iowa, Louisiana, Minnesota, Missouri, Montana, Nebraska, New York, North Carolina, Pennsylvania, Texas and Washington. *Child Maltreatment 2008 and 2009*, U.S. Department of Health and Human Services, Administration for Children and Families, Administration on Children, Youth and Families, Children's Bureau. 2009 and 2010.

[25] Burstain JM. *The 2012-13 Budget for Child Protective Services: The Good, the Bad and the Ugly.* Center for Public Policy Priorities. July 2011.

[26] Burstain JM. *The 2012-13 Budgetfor Child Protective Services: The Good, the Bad and the Ugly.* Center for Public Policy Priorities. July 2011.

[27] Alabama (18.5%), Alaska (29.2%), Colorado (26.2%), Connecticut (26.6%), Florida (22.5%), Maine (28.8%), Tennessee (29.5%) *Child Maltreatment 2009*, U.S. Department of Health and Human Services, Administration for Children and Families, Administration on Children, Youth and Families, Children's Bureau. 2009.

[28] Alaska, California, Colorado, Iowa, Montana, Nebraska, North Carolina, and Texas

[29] *Child Maltreatment 2009*, U.S. Department of Health and Human Services, Administration for Children and Families, Administration on Children, Youth and Families, Children's Bureau. 2009.

[30] Howard KS, Brooks-Gunn J. *The Role of Home-Visiting Programs in Preventing Child Abuse and Neglect.* Future of Children 19(2):1 19-146. Fall 2009.

[31] Burstain Testimony to the U.S. Senate Committee on Finance at the hearing on Innovations in Child Welfare Waivers: Starting the Pathway to Reform, March 10, 2011, at *http://cppp.org/files/4/Burstain* TitleIVWaiver SenateFinance.pdf(accessed July 8,2011).

[32] Waldfogel J. *Prevention and the Child Protective System.* Future of Children, 19(2):195-210. Fall 2009.

[33] Waldfogel J. *Prevention and the Child Protective System.* Future of Children, 19(2):195-210. Fall 2009.

[34] Texas Department of Family and Protective Services Legislative Appropriations Request for 2012-13.

[35] Based on what was expended for 2010 and estimated for 2011 versus what was appropriated in 2012-13.

[36] Base on the difference between what the state child welfare agency estimated it needed and what was actually funded. Burstain JM. *The 2012-13 Budgetfor Child Protective Services: The Good, the Bad and the Ugly.* Center for Public Policy Priorities. July 2011.

[37] Based on the Legislative Appropriations Requests of the Texas Workforce Commission and the Texas Department of Family and Protective Services.

[38] Wulczyn F. *Epidemiological Perspectives on Maltreatment Prevention.* Future of Children 1 9(2):39-66. Fall 2009.

[39] Wulczyn F. *Epidemiological Perspectives on Maltreatment Prevention.* Future of Children 1 9(2):39-66. Fall 2009.

[40] Mullick M, Miller LJ, Jacobsen T. *Insight Into Mental Illness and Child Maltreatment Risk Among Mothers with Major Psychiatric Disorder*. Psychiatric Services 52(4): 488-492. April 2001.

[41] Castro ED, Dunkelberg A, Pogue S, Mccown FS. *The Health Care Primer.* Center for Public Policy Priorities. 2011.

[42] Dunkelberg A, Pogue S. *Texas Health Reform Checklist: Key Steps to Make the Most of Reform.* Center for Public Policy Priorities. September 2010.

[43] Mullick M, Miller LJ, Jacobsen T. *Insight Into Mental Illness and Child Maltreatment Risk Among Mothers with Major Psychiatric Disorder*. Psychiatric Services 52(4): 488-492. April 2001.

INDEX

F

G

H

O

P

Q

R

S

T